Praise for *Your Cancer Road Map*

"While directing the series *The Emperor of All Maladies*, I was struck by all that we are learning about cancer at the cellular and molecular levels, and encouraged by the many exciting scientific advances we are witnessing. While this progress is cause for optimism, we cannot forget that thousands of lives across our country are disrupted by a diagnosis of cancer every single day. A disease as complex as cancer deserves a guidebook as comprehensive as *Your Cancer Road Map*. This candid, accessible approach to navigating cancer is the tonic every cancer patient needs."

—Barak Goodman, acclaimed nonfiction filmmaker and director of *Cancer: The Emperor of All Maladies*

"Cancer has affected so many close friends and family members, and they are the inspiration behind my philanthropic commitment to the Cancer Support Community. *Your Cancer Road Map* puts in one place the gold standard of innovative, patient-focused services and guidance that I am proud to have helped expand across the United States and to underserved communities. It is truly a gift to be a part of such a transformative and effective organization."

—Barbara Bradley Baekgaard, cofounder of Vera Bradley

"Kim Thiboldeaux is a fierce advocate for people living with cancer. I have known Kim and have had the privilege to collaborate with the Cancer Support Community for more than fifteen years and applaud their evidence-informed approach to patient care. *Your Cancer Road Map* is the guide that every cancer patient needs to relieve the stress of diagnosis and provide guidance and companionship throughout the cancer journey."

—Lidia Schapira, MD, FASCO, director of the Cancer Survivorship Program at the Stanford Cancer Institute

"As a husband who lost his wife to stage 4 lung cancer, I vowed to honor her memory by changing the face of lung cancer and raising awareness about the challenges survivors and their families face. As a former NFL linebacker, I understand the importance of a game plan, so I am committed to increasing the visibility of vital resources like *Your Cancer Road Map*. This comprehensive book reflects the intensely personal nature of the cancer experience and is a necessary resource for anyone confronting a cancer diagnosis. There is no one better prepared to give guidance and insight than Kim Thiboldeaux and the Cancer Support Community."

—Chris Draft, former NFL player and cofounder of Team Draft, an initiative of the Chris Draft Family Foundation

"The Cancer Support Community, led by Kim for the past twenty years, has been a great friend and partner to American Indians here in Arizona. They have supported our work to care for cancer patients on the Navajo Nation and have brought countless resources to our patients. *Your Cancer Road Map* is yet another example of the high quality of their work and their commitment to ensuring ALL people impacted by cancer have access to the highest-quality, culturally adapted cancer care and support."

—Lynette Bonar, RN, BSN, MBA, FACHE, CEO of Tuba City Regional Health Care Corporation

YOUR
CANCER
ROAD MAP

ALSO BY KIM THIBOLDEAUX

Reclaiming Your Life After Diagnosis: The Cancer Support Community Handbook (2012)

YOUR
CANCER
ROAD MAP

NAVIGATING LIFE WITH RESILIENCE

KIM THIBOLDEAUX

BenBella Books, Inc.
Dallas, TX

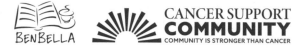

BenBella Books, Inc.
10440 N. Central Expressway
Suite 800
Dallas, TX 75231
www.benbellabooks.com
Send feedback to feedback@benbellabooks.com

BenBella is a federally registered trademark.

Printed in the United States of America
10 9 8 7 6 5 4 3 2 1

Library of Congress Control Number: 2020056662
ISBN 9781950665914 (trade paper)
ISBN 9781953295347 (electronic)

Editing by Jamie Kudera
Copyediting by Jennifer Greenstein
Proofreading by Christine Florie and Michael Fedison
Medical review by Craig Cole, MD
Indexing by IndexBusters
Text design and composition by PerfecType, Nashville, TN
Cover design by Faceout Studio, Molly von Borstel
Cover image © Shutterstock / christographcrowens
Printed by Versa Press
See interior image credits on page 285.

This book is dedicated to all people impacted by cancer.
May you find strength, healing, and hope.

CONTENTS

SECTION TWO
ACTIVE TREATMENT

SECTION THREE
AFTER TREATMENT IS DONE

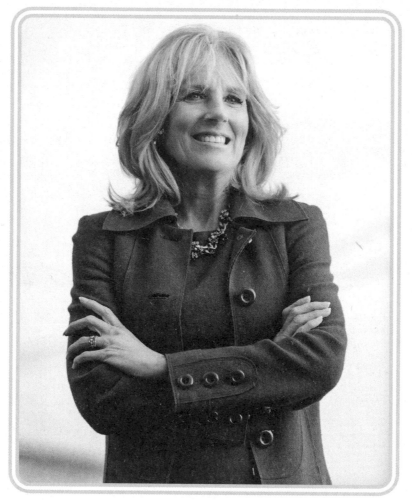

Photo by Ece Ogulturk

FOREWORD

Jill Biden

Growing up the oldest of five girls in a suburb of Philadelphia, I always wanted to be strong like my mother. She knew who she was—she was kind, self-possessed, always ready with the right words to say, and never someone to be carried away by her emotions. I wanted to be the person who was strong for everyone.

As a teacher of writing, my students often confide in me. They call me when they are distraught, and share their triumphs. I have felt lucky to be strong for them when they needed me.

A few years ago, however, I had to tell my class that I would miss the next session for personal reasons. By that point in the term, we had all become close, and no one seemed to have any real filters anymore. They all began shouting, "Where are you going, Dr. B.?" I told them, "My sister Jan is having a stem cell transplant. Today is her first treatment, and she'll have to stay in the same hospital room for six weeks." Standing there in front of the class, however, I could feel my resolve break and I suddenly lost my composure. I had to pause, as the next words caught in my throat. "I just . . . need to be with her."

I quickly faced the whiteboard so the students wouldn't see the tears filling my eyes. When I turned back around, every single student was standing. They made a line and came up to hug me, one by one.

Until that moment, I hadn't realized just how much I needed *their* strength.

Cancer has been a dark thread that has run through my life, as it has for so many Americans. In just one year, I watched four friends struggle with breast cancer. Cancer took the lives of both my parents. My son—my brave, funny, bright young son Beau—fought an excruciating fight against glioblastoma for over a year before we lost him.

Though medicine continues to advance and hope grows every year, there is still no word as frightening as *malignant*. No one should have to go through it alone. We can't; we need our community to support us. That's true for families and caregivers of patients as well.

That's why this book and Kim's voice are so critical.

When I met Kim Thiboldeaux, right away, I knew we would be friends. We are so alike in the ways that matter: both one of five kids, both Philly girls, both Eagles fans. More than that, though, we are both passionate about helping cancer patients and their families get the support they need—and ending this disease as we know it.

When Kim served on the Biden Cancer Initiative's board of directors, I saw her leadership in full force, driving progress and facilitating groundbreaking partnerships. In 2019, we visited the Navajo Nation in Arizona together to see the realization of that work, the opening of the first-ever full-time cancer care and support center on an American Indian reservation.

Kim understands how difficult the cancer journey can be—not just because patients face sickness and even death, but because a cancer diagnosis is a door to a complicated and foreign world. Patients and their families must navigate complex insurance and payment systems, learn obscure medical terms, understand complicated treatments, advocate for their health, and have difficult conversations with the people they love. And they must do it all without a road map or guide to show them the way. Until now.

It doesn't matter how strong you are. We all need people to lean on at times. A hug, a kind word, a steady voice, or a piece of advice—sometimes they are the lifelines that get us to the other side of anxiety and despair. I hope Kim's experience, wisdom, stories, and strength can be a lifeline through your journey. I hope this book reminds you that you are not alone.

INTRODUCTION

Over the past twenty-five years, I have talked to and met with thousands of cancer patients and their loved ones across the country and around the world. Among them are complete strangers and people who have known me since I was a child. They include friends, colleagues, neighbors, and contemporaries, some who are here today and some gone too soon.

Every story is different, unique, and personal. Yet over the years, I began to see common threads through each narrative. Each represents a life disrupted, a fear of the unknown, a desire for hope. Each person wants to feel confident in seeing the right doctors and making the right decisions. And each yearns for more time to fulfill unrealized dreams and aspirations.

I am often thrust into a stranger's life at their most difficult and vulnerable moments. I see each of these interactions as a privilege—a delicate thing to be cherished and safeguarded. I often say I have a front-row seat to the triumph of the human spirit. And in the end, I have received more from these exchanges than I have given.

This book is written to be a trusted ally for anyone diagnosed with cancer. It is called *Your Cancer Road Map* because it carefully and thoughtfully plots out the journey from start to finish. It includes instructions for navigating detours and warning signs, and tips to take in the scenery along the way, perhaps through a different lens. You'll encounter men—and women—at work, U-turns, and speed bumps. And also roadblocks, which can be discouraging and frustrating. Ultimately, this book is intended to shine a light and give you the tools and resources to find your way. I often say to folks, "There isn't a right way to take on cancer—there is only the way that is right for you. You're in the driver's seat and you will decide which road to take and how you choose to get to your desired destination."

The subtitle of the book is *Navigating Life with Resilience*. I have thought a great deal about resilience lately. What is resilience? How does one find it within oneself? Can it be discovered and assimilated from inspiration around us? I believe resilience comes with heightened self-awareness and an ability to embrace change and let go of the things that are out of our control. Resilience is like a muscle that needs exercise and strengthening. Becoming resilient takes practice—and patience. And building these skills will enhance your ability to recover and move forward.

I encourage you to write notes in the margins of this book, circle and highlight things that capture your attention or resonate with you, and dog-ear the pages. Keep it in your purse or briefcase or backpack and take it with you to doctor's appointments and chemo infusions. Read it in the late hours in bed or in the backyard with a cup of coffee. You can read a chapter here and there and put the book down to revisit later. Read it again when you need tips or resources. Pass it along to a spouse or friend to peruse.

My hope is that you use the tools in this book to become more resilient and more empowered as you face cancer. And I hope that you find grace and fortitude along the way and that you share our belief that community is stronger than cancer.

Visit the companion website to discover more about topics discussed in *Your Cancer Road Map*, find easy access to resources, and get to know author, Kim Thiboldeaux. cancersupportcommunity.org/YourCancerRoadMap

JUST DIAGNOSED

CHAPTER 1

Take a Deep Breath

You've just been diagnosed with cancer. Or maybe you just learned that your loved one has cancer. Take a deep breath. You're not alone—approximately 4,931 people will be diagnosed with cancer today and around 1.8 million people this year. As the comedian Gilda Radner once said, "Having cancer gave me membership in an elite club I'd rather not belong to."

In 2020, the United States saw a decrease in the number of deaths from cancer. At the same time, there was an increase in the number of cancers diagnosed. In other words, even as doctors are getting better at detecting and treating it, cancer is on the rise. Many people don't realize that the greatest risk factor for cancer is age. And with 77 million baby boomers in the United States, this increase is to be expected.

These numbers tell us a little about the larger story, but this book is about you. How are you . . . *really*? It is normal to feel sad, upset, worried, or anxious during this time. In fact, there are studies that say that many people with cancer—any type of cancer—feel the same three things when they first learn they have it. They feel a loss of control, a loss of hope, and a sense of isolation.

This is why it's important now to take a step back. Even though it may be hard, take a step back so you can start to move forward. The coming weeks and months, in all likelihood, will be overwhelming and scary—a roller-coaster ride. You will face decisions you never thought you'd have to make. How do I tell my kids I have cancer? How will this affect my family's finances? Will I be able to work? Should I consider a clinical trial? Am I going to be in pain? Will I die?

The good news? There are many national and local experts, organizations, and resources to help you through this journey. There are also services available at your hospital or clinic. You don't have to face cancer alone.

"When you're given a diagnosis, take a deep breath and say,
I can do this. I can deal with this.'"
—Carmen, lung cancer survivor

Now is a good time to center yourself. Think about what is important to you. This is also the time to think about how you want to face cancer. We all approach life and its challenges differently. For example, are you an information seeker—the kind of person who wants all the details, options, and alternatives? Or are you someone who wants less information and would prefer to leave decisions to your medical team? Are you a person who wants to keep everyone in your life up-to-date on your diagnosis and treatment, or are you more private? There is no one right way to approach cancer—only a right way for *you*.

As you begin to move forward, consider the ten tips for living well with cancer that appear at the end of this chapter. This list comes from *Frankly Speaking About Cancer*, an award-winning educational series by the Cancer Support Community (CSC). You will see many references in this book to CSC's *Frankly Speaking* materials, which are available for free on our website at www.cancersupportcommunity.org.

These tips can help you create a plan and framework for facing cancer. Remember, you are not alone as you go down this road. Rely on friends and family, your health care team, advocacy organizations, and community resources. They can provide answers, support, and guidance on all aspects of your treatment, care, and well-being.

"Don't read or believe everything you see on the internet. Surround yourself with positive people. Join a support group. Breathe. Everything's going to be okay."
—Lynn, chronic lymphocytic leukemia survivor

Excerpt from *Why Did I Come into This Room? A Candid Conversation About Aging*

JOAN LUNDEN

An award-winning journalist, bestselling author, motivational speaker, and women's health and wellness advocate, Joan Lunden has been a trusted voice in American homes for more than forty years. Lunden documented her battle through breast cancer treatment and wrote a candid and poignant memoir, Had I Known, *about her experience.*

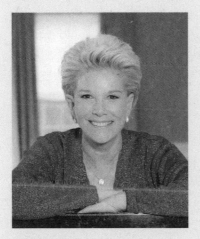

Photo by Daphne Youree

It's not easy telling people that you have cancer, or any other serious disease for that matter. For me, it felt like I was flawed, no longer a healthy, vibrant individual. I remember sitting in the salon the day I got my head shaved. I wanted to feel like GI Joan but when I looked in the mirror, no getting around it, I looked like a cancer patient.

With some reservation at the outset, I decided to go public with my diagnosis in the hopes that it might give me the opportunity to make an important impact on women's health. You know that saying, "The truth will set you free"? Well, that was certainly the case for me. As soon as I took my story wide, the breast cancer community reached out to me to speak around the country. I began documenting and sharing my cancer battle online. I finally felt like I was becoming a real warrior in my battle. This public campaign shifted my mental focus from my own personal cancer to the fight against all cancer.

It's been said that helping others helps yourself. This was certainly true for me. My advocacy changed my breast cancer journey in the most positive way and my life was starting to take on a whole new purpose. As I was battling my cancer, I was helping others. I once read that when you overcome loss, you gain new strength. I just hoped I was as strong as everyone kept saying I was.

I traveled the country sharing what I'd learned on my journey. I went to Washington, DC, and knocked on senators' doors to lobby for needed changes in health care policy. I had found a new community, the breast cancer community, and I was awestruck by the power and sense of loyalty that this unique sorority had. No matter where I went, whether to a conference, a breast cancer awareness luncheon, or to a Pink Run/Walk, it seemed that every female member was instinctually reaching out and checking on other women there, lending their advice or simply their strength.

Those wonderful women made me a better person. They taught me to more fully give of myself. They instilled in me a deeper, resounding compassion for each and every woman who walks our path. They made me more resilient. They helped me to believe I would beat my cancer, that I would make it over the finish line. And I did. I'm happy to report that after sixteen rounds of aggressive chemo, as well as surgery and six weeks of radiation, I remain cancer free.

RESOURCES TO HELP YOU GET STARTED

Cancer Support Community's "Cancer Diagnosis? What You Need to Know"—Content and links to helpful resources to address concerns and questions that arise at diagnosis. www.CancerSupportCommunity.org/cancer-diagnosis-what-you-need-know

Cancer Support Community's *Frankly Speaking About Cancer: Making Treatment Decisions*—A must-read for patients on the verge of making treatment decisions. www.CancerSupportCommunity.org/make-treatment-decision-right-you

Cancer Support Community's "Tips for Newly Diagnosed"—Tips and video advice from people who have been where you are now. www.cancersupportcommunity.org /tips-newly-diagnosed

TEN TIPS FOR LIVING WELL WITH CANCER*

TAKE ONE STEP AT A TIME, AND MAKE ONE DECISION AT A TIME

If life feels overwhelming, take small steps to find your best path. Talk, listen, and learn. In time, you will have the information you need to make the right decisions for you.

PAY ATTENTION TO WHAT YOU NEED

Be aware of your feelings. Focus on activities you enjoy. Try to find humor in each day. Seek out people who help you feel relaxed or happy. Spend time alone if you need to. Some days you may not know what you need, and that's okay, too. **Be kind to yourself.**

BE YOUR OWN BEST ADVOCATE

You may feel frustrated by changes to your life. Talk with your medical team and your family and friends. Work together to come up with a plan that gives you as much control as possible over your treatment and care.

COMMUNICATE EFFECTIVELY WITH YOUR HEALTH CARE TEAM

Let your health care team know how you feel. Ask questions and ask again if you don't understand the answers. Tell your team about your goals for treatment. Be sure they know how your treatment and symptoms are affecting your everyday life.

GET HELP FROM OTHERS, BESIDES YOUR DOCTOR

Expand your health care team to include a patient advocate and other specialists. A patient advocate or navigator can help you find resources, manage insurance, and prepare legal documents. Other useful specialists may include a nutritionist to help with eating, a psychologist or social worker for emotional distress, a physical therapist for weakness, and a palliative care specialist for symptom management.

MAINTAIN HOPE

Hope can make each day a little better. Accept that some days will be better than others, but try to enjoy small moments and do things that make you smile. Even if a cure is unlikely, look for ways to find hope where you can.

REACH OUT TO OTHERS WITH CANCER

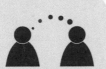

It's comforting to talk with people who understand what you're going through. Try to connect with others online or in a local support group.

ASK FOR SUPPORT AND ACCEPT HELP WHEN IT IS OFFERED

Let your family and friends know how they can support you. Be specific if you can. Consider using an online platform and calendar such as the Cancer Support Community's MyLifeLine to stay organized and let friends know what's needed.

FOCUS ON NUTRITION, EXERCISE, AND MIND-BODY WELLNESS

Healthy food provides nutrients to help your body. Exercise can lift your spirits, boost your energy, and reduce stress. Meditation and mindfulness can bring a sense of calm. Even minor efforts can help you feel better.

KEEP A NOTEBOOK NEARBY

Use a notebook to keep track of side effects, take notes when you talk with your health care team, and record financial or insurance details.

*Adapted from Cancer Support Community, *Frankly Speaking About Cancer: Metastatic Breast Cancer*, February 2019, www.cancersupportcommunity.org/sites/default/files/fields/resource/file/2018-03/mbc_book_2018.pdf.

CHAPTER 2

Know Your Diagnosis and Stage of Disease

We sometimes think of cancer as one disease. But, in fact, there are hundreds of different types and subtypes of cancer. Each requires its own approach to diagnosis and treatment.

When you are diagnosed with cancer, one of the most important things you can do is to learn about the kind of cancer you have. Start by gathering as much information as possible about your specific type of cancer and the stage of disease. You can do this in two ways:

- *Talk with your health care team.* Your doctor can tell you the type, subtype, and stage of disease. Ask about both genetic (mutation) testing and biomarker testing, which we will discuss in chapter five. Your health care team can provide this information and explain what it means. You can also ask for a copy of your pathology report and any other lab or test results. A pathology report is written by a pathologist, a scientist who studies disease. In cancer, this is the doctor who looks at your cells and tissues under a microscope. Their report helps determine your exact diagnosis. All this information drives the decision-making process.

- *Refer to trusted sources.* Use the resources in this book and on the Cancer Support Community's website to find the names of trusted websites and organizations where you can learn more about specific cancers. Your health care team can also recommend resources. Cancer is complex. You will learn a lot quickly. The more you learn, the more confident you will feel making treatment decisions.

DIAGNOSIS

The first step is to understand how your doctor has determined that you have cancer. Here are some ways that cancer may be diagnosed:

Biopsy: The removal of cells or tissues for examination by a pathologist to see whether cancer is present. The pathologist may study the tissue under a microscope or perform other tests on the cells or tissue.[1]

Blood test: A test done on a sample of blood to measure the amount of certain substances in the blood or to count different types of blood cells. Blood tests may be used to look for signs of disease or agents that cause disease, to check for antibodies or tumor markers, or to see how well treatments are working.[2]

Bone scan: An imaging procedure that uses a radioactive tracer to look for cancer or other changes in the bone.[3]

Computerized tomography (CT) scan: A series of detailed pictures of areas inside the body, taken from different angles. The pictures are created by a computer linked to an X-ray machine. This is also called a CAT scan.[4]

---

1. Cancer Support Community, *Frankly Speaking About Cancer: Metastatic Breast Cancer*, February 2019, www.cancersupportcommunity.org/mbc.

2. NCI Dictionary of Cancer Terms, National Cancer Institute, accessed October 19, 2020, www.cancer.gov/publications/dictionaries/cancer-terms.

3. Cancer Support Community, *Frankly Speaking: Metastatic Breast Cancer.*

4. Cancer Support Community, *Frankly Speaking: Metastatic Breast Cancer.*

Magnetic resonance imaging (MRI): A procedure in which radio waves and a powerful magnet linked to a computer are used to create detailed pictures of areas inside the body. These pictures can show the difference between normal and diseased tissue.[5]

Positron emission tomography (PET) scan: A procedure in which a small amount of radioactive glucose (sugar) is injected into a vein, and a scanner is used to make detailed, computerized pictures of areas inside the body where the glucose is used. It is used to detect the location of cancers in parts of the body, where cancer cells use more glucose than normal cells.[6]

Ultrasound: A procedure that uses high-energy sound waves to look at tissues and organs inside the body. The sound waves make echoes that form pictures of the tissues and organs on a computer screen (sonogram).[7]

As your health care team diagnoses your cancer, they will also determine the stage and grade of your disease. Each cancer type is staged or graded differently. The purpose of staging is to find out if your cancer is confined to one area or if it has spread beyond the initial site to other parts of the body. Grade focuses more on how the cells look under a microscope.

Knowing the stage or grade of your cancer will guide the treatment plan. It will also inform the goals of therapy. For example, if your cancer is in an early stage and has not spread to other parts of the body, the goal of treatment may be to eliminate the cancer completely. If the cancer has spread to other parts of the body, the goal may be to shrink the tumor or slow the spread of disease.

STAGING

Let's take a look at a couple of examples of how cancer is staged. One of the most commonly used standards is the TNM staging system.[8] It is used for most solid

---

5. NCI Dictionary of Cancer Terms.

6. NCI Dictionary of Cancer Terms.

7. NCI Dictionary of Cancer Terms.

8. The TNM staging system was developed and is maintained by the American Joint Committee on Cancer and the Union for International Cancer Control. More information can be found at cancerstaging.org.

tumor cancers, including breast, colon, and non–small cell lung. TNM takes into consideration:

Tumor (T): How big is the tumor? Where is it located? Has it directly invaded nearby tissue?

Lymph nodes (N): Has the cancer spread to the lymph nodes in and around the tumor site?

Metastasis (M): Has the cancer spread to other parts of the body?

Doctors look at the TNM numbers as a group. Because of this, it is hard to describe the stages in just a few words. For example, the stages of non–small cell lung cancer are as follows:[9]

Stage 0 (carcinoma in situ): This is a very early stage, marked by abnormal cells only in the air passages.

Stages IA and IB (1A and 1B): At these stages, the tumor is small and cancer has not spread to the lymph nodes. In stage IA, the tumor is 3 centimeters (cm) or less. In stage IB, the tumor is between 3 and 4 cm.

Stages IIA and IIB (2A and 2B): In stage IIA, the tumor is between 4 and 5 cm. It has not spread to the lymph nodes. In stage IIB, the tumor is smaller than 5 cm and cancer has spread to the lymph nodes on the same side of the chest as the tumor.

Stages IIIA, IIIB, and IIIC (3A, 3B, and 3C): In these stages, the cancer has spread to the lymph nodes. It has not spread to other parts of the body. The tumor may be bigger, or the cancer may be in an area that is harder to reach than cancers in earlier stages. Stages IIIB and IIIC are often treated more like stage IV cancers.

Stage IV (4): In this stage, the cancer has spread beyond one lung. It is in the other lung, the fluid near the lung or heart, or another part of the body. When it spreads, lung cancer can go anywhere, but often spreads to the brain, bones, liver, or adrenal glands.

---

9. Cancer Support Community, *Frankly Speaking About Cancer: Lung Cancer*, June 2020, www .cancersupportcommunity.org/lungbook.

Staging varies among cancers, even when the same system is used. Breast cancer also uses the TNM staging system, but doctors make subtle distinctions among the T, N, and M measures. To give you a sense, T has thirteen different levels, including one for a tumor that cannot be evaluated (TX). In 2018, the stages were updated to include biomarkers in staging. In other words, the same stage of breast cancer can look and act in many different ways.

Blood cancers are staged differently. Doctors use the Lugano classification for non-Hodgkin lymphoma, a cancer that starts in the immune system. The stages look like this:[10]

Stage I: This stage is divided between I and IE. In I, cancer is found in one lymph node area (such as the tonsils). In stage IE, cancer is in one organ or one area outside the lymph system.

Stage II: This stage uses the diaphragm, in the middle of the body, as a divider. The cancer is confined to either the top or bottom of the body. Cancer is found in two or more areas, either on top of or below the diaphragm. In IIE, cancer may be in one lymph node area and a nearby organ and the lymph nodes around it. It may also affect groups of lymph nodes on the same side of the diaphragm.

Stage III: Cancer is found in lymph nodes both above and below the diaphragm or in the lymph nodes above the diaphragm and in the spleen.

Stage IV: The lymphoma has spread widely into at least one organ outside the lymph system, such as the bone marrow, liver, or lung.

GRADING

When cancer starts in the brain, another approach is taken. Unlike lung cancer, brain tumors are graded using a system from the World Health Organization. The grade describes how the cells look under a microscope. Cells that look more abnormal grow and spread faster. Let's take a look at the grades and what they mean:[11]

10. "Non-Hodgkin Lymphoma Stages," American Cancer Society, last revised August 1, 2018, www.cancer.org/cancer/non-hodgkin-lymphoma/detection-diagnosis-staging/staging.html.

11. National Cancer Institute, "Adult Central Nervous System Tumors Treatment (PDQ)," accessed March 13, 2021, www.cancer.gov/types/brain/patient/adult-brain-treatment-pdq.

Grade I: The cells look normal and are unlikely to spread or grow. They usually can be removed by surgery.

Grade II: The cells look a little less normal than in grade I. They are still slow to grow and spread. After treatment, the tumor may come back at a higher grade.

Grade III: The cells look even more abnormal and may spread to other parts of the brain. The tumor is likely to come back at a higher grade.

Grade IV: The tumor is fast growing. The cells look very abnormal and easily spread within the brain.

After your cancer is staged or graded, you will spend time with you doctor discussing possible treatment plans and other next steps, which we will go over in chapter four.

"The only way we could get any control was to get information. From the beginning, that is the approach we've taken: what do we know, what don't we know, what are the possibilities."

—Richard, ocular melanoma survivor

RESOURCES ON DIAGNOSIS AND STAGE OF DISEASE

These four organizations maintain updated content on cancer diagnosis and treatment, including disease staging. Enter the type of cancer on their home page and go from there. Disease-specific websites can be good resources as well. Refer to the resources at the end of this book for a more complete list of where to go for education and support.

American Cancer Society—www.cancer.org
American Society of Clinical Oncology—www.cancer.net
Cancer Support Community—www.cancersupportcommunity.org
National Cancer Institute—www.cancer.gov

CHAPTER 3

Build Your Team

As the news of a cancer diagnosis sets in, you will have many medical appointments. Take time to prepare so you can get the most out of every conversation.

DON'T DO IT ALONE

We strongly recommend bringing a friend or family member to all your appointments. This person can be a second set of ears. They can help take notes and clarify information. Sometimes the sheer emotion of a cancer diagnosis can interfere with our thinking. It can be difficult to listen to health information and keep a clear head. This is where a loved one comes in. They can help ensure that you walk away with the information you need to process what you've heard and think about next steps.

It is important, however, to take the *right* person with you for these appointments. Some people like to bring more than one person, which is also fine. It is logical, for example, to bring a spouse or partner along. That person, however, may be as emotionally affected as you are by the diagnosis. Consider someone who is a careful listener and good notetaker. Find a person who will respect your priorities and values today, and as you move forward.

Discuss with this person in advance the role you are hoping for them to play. Let them know, for example, if they are there just to take notes or if they can assist in other ways. Would it be helpful if they asked questions? Let them know if you want them in the room for only part of the appointment. You may want some one-on-one time with the doctor for more private or sensitive matters. It may be useful to review with the person beforehand the list of questions and topics you want to cover.

In this chapter, we share some questions to ask as you look for the right doctor. In chapter six, we will discuss decision-making and offer suggestions for other questions to ask now and at critical points in the future.

"Bring that notetaker because you will be surprised. As much as you think you are intelligent and you've got it all together, you will not remember something, or you and your spouse will remember it differently."
—Mariann, breast cancer survivor and former lung cancer caregiver

---

KEY QUESTIONS FOR THE DOCTOR[1]

These questions can help you decide who your doctor will be. A doctor should feel comfortable answering these questions. If they do not want to answer them, find another doctor who will.

- How much experience do you (the doctor) have in treating this specific type of cancer?
- Are you board certified in medical, surgical, and/or radiation oncology?

---

1. "Caregivers," Cancer Support Community, accessed November 16, 2020, www
.cancersupportcommunity.org/caregivers.

- Are you and your team up-to-date on the latest treatments for this type of cancer? What are the most recent advances? Do you conduct clinical trials here to treat the kind of cancer I have?
- Do you and the hospital where treatment will be provided accept my insurance?
- Do you have an oncology nurse and/or oncology social worker on staff to provide me with education and support?
- What other support services are available?
- How and when can we contact you or other members of the cancer team with ongoing questions? (Can we use email? Talk to you on the phone? Or will we only be able to talk to you directly during office visits?)
- Can you give us the name of another oncologist, for a second opinion?

"It's a whole team. It's not just the doctor. Everyone has to be good at their jobs and you have to trust the whole group."
—Laura, multiple myeloma survivor

THE TEAM

As you begin down this road, you will see a team start to form around you. Your team may include your caregiver and others. Some members of the team are there because of your specific diagnosis and cancer center, and some are brought on by you. Each member of your health care team will take care of you in a different way. Here are some people who may be on your team and a bit about their roles:[2]

---

2. Cancer Support Community, *Frankly Speaking About Cancer: Metastatic Breast Cancer*, February 2019, www.cancersupportcommunity.org/mbc.

Medical oncologist: Diagnoses and treats cancer. They will oversee your treatment. Try to find one who focuses on the kind of cancer you have. For common cancers, this means someone whose practice is at least 50 percent dedicated to treatment of this cancer.

Hematologist: Diagnoses and treats blood cancers like leukemia, lymphoma, and multiple myeloma. Many medical oncologists also have training and are board certified in hematology.

Primary care physician: See this doctor for regular checkups and non-cancer-related issues like diabetes, hypertension, or asthma.

Oncology nurse practitioner (NP) / oncology physician assistant (PA): Can diagnose and treat medical problems and prescribe medicine. They may see you with your doctor or independently. This may be the person you contact with urgent questions or concerns.

Oncology nurse: A registered nurse (RN) who specializes in cancer. Often, they administer treatments and other medicines. They can help you understand your cancer diagnosis and treatment. They can be a good source of information and support.

Surgical oncologist: If surgery is recommended, look for a surgeon who specializes in that surgery. Ask how many times they have done that operation.

Radiation oncologist: Will manage any radiation treatments.

Radiologist: Oversees the scans used to diagnose and monitor you, including ultrasound, X-ray, MRI, CT scan, bone scan, and PET scan.

Palliative care specialist: Helps manage symptoms, pain, and side effects.

Oncology social worker: Can provide counseling. They can also help you with financial, transportation, and home care needs.

Psychologist/psychiatrist: Both can provide mental health care to support you before, during, or after treatment. A psychiatrist can also prescribe medicine.

Nutritionist/registered dietitian: Can help find foods to eat or ways to eat them to provide the nutrients you need. Look for a registered dietician (RDN) who has experience working with people with cancer.

Patient navigator/nurse navigator: Can help you talk with your health care team, help set up appointments, and help you get financial, legal, and social support.

Physical therapist/rehabilitation medical therapist: Can help treat physical discomfort that interferes with daily life. Some are certified in cancer.

Oncology pharmacist: Has special training in cancer medicines. They can teach you about drugs and how they interact. They can help you manage side effects. They also may help you find co-pay assistance or discounts.

Chaplain: Can offer emotional and spiritual support. You also may find support from clergy outside the hospital.

Try to collect and keep business cards from the members of your team. Ask them for the best way to reach them with any questions or concerns. Dealing with many people may feel overwhelming, but having a diverse and skilled team of specialists will ensure that you get the care and advice you need.

"When I was diagnosed, an incredible team came together with one goal—to save my life. Becoming knowledgeable about my disease, course of treatment, and what I could do for myself was the best thing I could do to be an active part of my team and help us reach our common goal."

—Andy, acute myeloid leukemia survivor

RESOURCES TO HELP YOU GET STARTED BUILDING YOUR TEAM

American Society of Clinical Oncology Find a cancer doctor on the website of the world's largest professional organization for medical oncologists. www.cancer.net /find-cancer-doctor

Cancer Support Community's "Caregivers"—Information and resources to get started when someone you love has cancer. www.cancersupportcommunity.org/caregivers

Cancer Support Community's *Frankly Speaking About Cancer: Making Treatment Decisions*—A must-read for patients on the verge of making treatment decisions. www.CancerSupportCommunity.org/make-treatment-decision-right-you

National Cancer Institute (NCI)—Find a multidisciplinary care team at an NCI-designated comprehensive cancer center, a hospital or cancer center in the United States recognized for leading cancer research and care. www.cancer.gov/research/nci-role/cancer-centers/find

CHAPTER 4

Understand Your Treatment Options

Once your cancer has been diagnosed and staged, your doctor will begin to discuss a treatment plan with you. There are many ways to treat cancer. Your treatment plan may include one, two, or more forms of treatment. You may have them at the same time or one right after the other. For example, you might have surgery and chemotherapy, or radiation and immunotherapy. Or you might have a combination of drugs, including chemotherapy and immunotherapy.

Your doctor will recommend treatment based on what they have learned about your cancer. They will match this information with the accepted guidelines for the type of cancer you have. These guidelines are issued by expert panels and reviewers. Doctors also call this the *standard of care* or *best practice guidelines*.

Let's take a minute to talk about the guidelines. In the United States, two key groups issue guidelines for cancer treatment:

- *The National Comprehensive Cancer Network (NCCN)* is made up of some of the top cancer centers in the United States. Its treatment guidelines address every disease and stage. The guidelines focus on treatment and follow-up. NCCN relies on published data but also gathers consensus from leading doctors and hospitals. These guidelines are easy to find and widely used.
- *The American Society of Clinical Oncology (ASCO)* also puts out clinical practice guidelines. ASCO is the professional society of cancer doctors in the United States. Its guidelines are also based on published data. They take into account the methods used in the studies. They offer advice on "a single question or a group of questions around an important topic."[1]

Doctors also consult with each other before recommending treatment. When a case is complex or there are many options for treatment, a doctor may bring it to the hospital or cancer center's tumor board. A tumor board consists of doctors, nurses, and other experts in the treatment of cancer. They look at cases together and discuss recommendations. The shared wisdom and experience of the multidisciplinary group can shed light on the best path forward. Your doctor may also talk with doctors from other hospitals. Or you may choose to do that yourself. In chapter seven, we will discuss getting a second opinion.

———————————

"Take a deep breath and ask questions. Become your own advocate.
Ask for information and know the right questions to ask your health care team.
This is really important when deciding on a treatment plan. Especially ask about
the short- and long-term effects of any treatment."
—Dave, head and neck cancer survivor

———————————

It is important that you, too, are an active member of your health care team. Learn about your treatment options so you are prepared to take on cancer as a fully informed

———————————

1. Mark R. Somerfield, Karen L. Hagerty, and Christopher E. Desch, "ASCO Clinical Practice Guidelines: Frequently Asked Questions," *Journal of Oncology Practice* 2, no. 1 (2006): 41–43.

partner in your own care. Let's take a look at some of the most common treatments for cancer:[2]

Surgery: Surgery is an operation to remove the cancer (or part of it) from your body. It is not always possible or helpful. When it is thought that the cancer can be completely removed, surgery is often the first treatment. The most common side effects are pain, fatigue, bleeding, swelling around the surgical site, and infection.

Chemotherapy: Chemotherapy (also called chemo) uses drugs to attack and kill cancer cells. These very strong drugs attack fast-growing cells like cancer. Chemo can cause side effects like hair loss, nausea, mouth sores, and low white blood cell counts.

Radiation therapy (radiotherapy): Radiation therapy uses strong energy beams, such as very strong X-rays, electrons, or protons, to kill cancer cells and shrink tumors. Radiation can also damage normal tissue or organs, so it is carefully focused to reduce that damage. You may experience redness, burns, or hair loss in the area being treated. Other possible side effects include fatigue, loss of appetite, and nausea.

Immunotherapy: Immunotherapy works by making the immune system stronger so it can fight cancer better. The immune system helps your body fight infections and other diseases, like cancer. But sometimes cancers learn how to avoid the immune system and grow anyway. Immunotherapy works to turn the immune system back on to fight the cancer. Common side effects include fatigue, skin problems, fever, and shortness of breath. Most side effects are mild, but some can be severe.

Targeted therapy: Targeted therapy targets specific changes in a gene or cell that cause cancers to grow, divide, or spread. Doctors test tumors for these changes (biomarkers) to find out if targeted therapy may work. Diarrhea and skin problems, including rashes, are the most common side effects.

Hormone therapy: Hormone therapy is the use of drugs to block hormones that drive cancer growth. It is used to treat cancers that rely on hormones to grow, such as

---

2. Definitions adapted from Cancer Support Community, *Frankly Speaking About Cancer: Targeted Therapy and Biomarker Testing for Lung Cancer,* August 2019, www.cancersupport community.org/targetedlung.

some breast and prostate cancers. Common side effects include tiredness, hot flashes, weight gain, and loss of bone density.

Stem cell transplant: Stem cell transplant is a procedure used to treat some blood cancers. It is a way to deliver high doses of chemotherapy and replace blood cells that have been destroyed by chemotherapy or radiation with fresh unharmed stem cells. Bone marrow transplant is one kind of stem cell transplant. Sometimes patients serve as their own donors (autologous stem cell transplant), and other times patients get stem cells from donors (allogeneic stem cell transplant). Doctors monitor transplant patients closely to avoid serious side effects such as very low blood counts and hard-to-treat infections.

Watch and wait: Your health care team may take this approach if there are minimal changes in your test results or blood counts and no symptoms. You will see a doctor regularly but won't begin treatment until needed. This is sometimes called watchful waiting or active surveillance.[3]

It is important to take time to understand the treatments that you will receive, how they will be given (e.g., by vein or by mouth), how often, and where. Ask lots of questions. Ask your doctor to write down the names of the drugs you will take and the doses. You will find that most drugs have a brand name and a generic name. Ask for both names so you have an accurate record. In chapter sixteen, we will talk about the side effects of cancer treatment and some tips for tracking and managing them.

"I was fortunate because everything went according to schedule. Before the procedure, the hospital had a meeting for everyone who would be getting a stem cell transplant. They tried to prepare us as much as possible. They told us what would happen every step of the way. That really helped."
—Laura, multiple myeloma survivor

---

3. "Active Surveillance," Cancer Support Community, accessed November 13, 2020, www.cancer supportcommunity.org/article/active-surveillance.

RESOURCES TO LEARN MORE ABOUT TREATMENT OPTIONS

American Cancer Society's "Treatment Types"—Learn more about cancer treatment approaches. www.cancer.org/treatment/treatments-and-side-effects/treatment-types .html

ASCO Care and Treatment Recommendations for Patients—Learn more about cancer treatment guidelines. www.cancer.net/research-and-advocacy/asco-care-and -treatment-recommendations-patients

ASCO Clinical Practice Guidelines—Look up specific ASCO guidelines by topic. www .asco.org/research-guidelines/quality-guidelines/guidelines

Cancer Support Community's "Cancer Treatment"—Tips to help with treatment planning and learn about specific cancers. www.cancersupportcommunity.org/cancer -treatment

National Cancer Institute's "Types of Cancer Treatment"—Learn more about cancer treatment approaches. www.canccr.gov/about-cancer/treatment/types

National Comprehensive Cancer Network Guidelines for Patients—Look up NCCN guidelines by type of cancer. www.nccn.org/patients/guidelines/cancers.aspx

CHAPTER 5

Learn About Genetic and Genomic Testing

I n this chapter, we will talk about the difference between genetics and genomics. These words are used quite often when we talk about cancer. They are sometimes used interchangeably but, in fact, have different meanings. We want to help you understand what they mean and what genetic and genomic tests can tell you about yourself, your risk of cancer, and the best treatment options for you. We will explain the differences between these terms and give examples of tests for each.

While we still don't know what causes most cancers, advances in science provide a window into how genes passed through families may make it more likely that we will develop some cancers. Likewise, we know more about how genes in our bodies change in our lifetimes and how some drive tumor growth. Both types of genes play a role in cancer.

GENETICS AND GENETIC TESTING

Let's start with genetics. Genetics, simply put, is the study of heredity. Heredity is the way traits are passed down through families. We inherit many traits and physical characteristics from our families. These can include the color of our eyes, the hand we use for writing, or even a temper! Doctors estimate that 5 to 10 percent of cancers are due to an inherited gene.[1]

You may be wondering if there's a way to find out if your family history increases your risk of cancer. Yes and no. In some cases, it makes sense to get tested for family cancer risk. But who should get tested? To answer this question, many doctors turn to the U.S. Preventive Services Task Force (USPSTF). The USPSTF is "an independent, volunteer panel of national experts in disease prevention and evidence-based medicine. The Task Force works to improve the health of all Americans by making evidence-based recommendations about clinical preventive services."[2] The task force is made up of sixteen volunteer members who are experts in their fields. They set guidelines for preventive screenings, tests, counseling, and medicines.

Doctors use these guidelines to decide when to recommend genetic testing. Most people who have cancer will not have a genetic test. Tests are done only when doctors suspect a genetic link and this information will affect treatment or the risk of other cancers. Doctors look for a family pattern, not just one person with cancer, before they suggest testing. This can be hard to accept, especially when you have a cancer that is known to run in families. But be assured that the guidelines are in place for a reason and are based on a significant amount of data. Reviewing the guidelines and talking with your doctor should lead to a shared decision that makes sense for you and your family.

Now let's look at the timing of testing. You may have been tested for a cancer gene before you had cancer. This test was offered to you because your family history suggested that you might have a higher risk of cancer. And, importantly, there was something you could do to reduce that risk.

If your doctor thinks that genetic testing may be useful, they may refer you to a genetic counselor. There may be one at the hospital or clinic where you are being treated. If not, they may refer you to one in your community. You can also find genetic counselors

---

1. "The Genetics of Cancer," National Cancer Institute, October 12, 2017, www.cancer.gov /about-cancer/causes-prevention/genetics#syndromes.

2. U.S. Preventive Services Task Force home page, accessed April 1, 2020, www.uspreventive servicestaskforce.org/uspstf/.

through the website of the National Society of Genetic Counselors (www.nsgc.org). A genetic counselor can help you:

- understand your test results and what they mean for you.
- understand what these results may mean for your family.
- make decisions about prevention, treatment, surveillance, and telling others.

Some people choose to see a genetic counselor before they are tested to discuss what they might do if they test positive. If you are considering this, check with your insurance company to find out if genetic counseling is covered under your plan.

Let's take a minute to look at one example of an inherited cancer. You may have heard of *BRCA1* or *BRCA2*. A change (often called a mutation) in the *BRCA* gene may increase your risk of breast and ovarian cancer. If you have one of these cancers, your doctor will likely ask you about your family history of cancer. Even if your doctor does not ask, it is important to tell them. Try to be as specific as you can. For each family member who had cancer, it is helpful to know:

- how the person is related to you.
- the kind of cancer they had.
- when they had cancer.
- how old they were when the cancer was diagnosed.

Your doctor will use this information to decide if the USPSTF guidelines call for testing. Many insurance companies will pay for testing only if it is indicated based on these guidelines.

Here are some other examples of hereditary cancer syndromes:

Cowden syndrome: A change in the *PTEN* gene causes benign (not cancer) growths to form. People with this syndrome have a higher risk of breast, thyroid, endometrial, and other cancers.

Hereditary breast and ovarian cancer syndrome: This is the *BRCA* example given above. In addition to a higher risk of breast and ovarian cancer, people with this syndrome may be more likely to have cancer of the fallopian tubes, prostate, or pancreas.

Li-Fraumeni syndrome: This rare syndrome often affects people when they are younger. It is caused by a change in the *TP53* gene. People who have this are more likely to develop leukemia or cancers of the bone, brain, breast, or adrenal glands (near the kidney). They may have more than one of these cancers in a lifetime. They also are more likely to get cancer as a result of radiation.

Lynch syndrome: This is also called hereditary non-polyposis colorectal cancer (HNPCC). People with Lynch syndrome have a much higher risk of colorectal cancer. They also may be more likely to develop these cancers: bile duct, breast, endometrial (uterine), kidney, liver, ovarian, pancreatic, prostate, small bowel, stomach, and urinary tract.

GENOMICS AND BIOMARKER TESTING

Now let's turn to genomics. Genomics is the scientific study of the complete set of DNA—all our genes. In cancer, genomic testing looks for changes (mutations) in the genes or cells of a person with cancer that may be causing cancer to grow and spread. You may hear this kind of testing referred to as molecular testing, next-generation sequencing (NGS), or biomarker testing. Testing is done on a sample of tumor tissue, which was removed during a biopsy, or on your blood. Testing your blood for these kinds of changes is called a liquid biopsy.

In this book, we will refer to genomic testing broadly as biomarker testing. Biomarkers are measurable signs of a change in a gene or cell. Today, doctors can order biomarker tests for a wide range of cancers, including lung cancer, breast cancer, colorectal cancer, and others. These tests are used to guide treatment. A positive test may open the door to more treatment options.

In the past several years, there have been notable scientific advances in biomarker testing for lung cancer. So let's use lung cancer as an example. Scientists have developed drugs to treat lung cancers with these biomarkers:[3]

---

3. Cancer Support Community, "Biomarker Testing for Lung Cancer Tool," www.cancersupport community.org/biomarker-testing-tool; Cancer Support Community, *Frankly Speaking About Cancer: Targeted Therapy and Biomarker Testing for Lung Cancer*, August 2019, www.cancersupport community.org/targetedlung.

ALK: ALK (anaplastic lymphoma kinase) is the gene that makes the ALK protein. ALK plays a role in cell growth. It can stop the growth of unhealthy cells. *ALK* can change and stop working. It may move or fuse to another gene. This is called *ALK* rearrangement. When this happens, cancer can grow. This is seen in some lung cancers, neuroblastomas, and lymphomas.

BRAF: BRAF is the gene that makes the BRAF protein. BRAF plays a role in cell signaling and cell growth. It can change and stop working. When this happens, BRAF sends signals that make cancer grow. This is seen in some melanomas and cancers of the lung, thyroid, ovaries, and colon.

EGFR: EGFR (epidermal growth factor receptor) is the gene that makes the EGFR protein. The protein is found on cells. It helps cells grow and divide. Cancer cells sometimes have too much EGFR, causing the disease to grow and spread.

MET: MET is the gene that makes the MET protein. It plays a role in cell signaling and cell growth. The *MET* gene can change and become amplified so it is stronger or there is more of it. When this happens, cancer can grow and spread. It is seen in some lung, liver, kidney, and head and neck cancers.

NTRK: NTRK (neurotrophic tyrosine receptor kinase) is a gene that can change and join with other genes. This is called *NTRK* gene fusion. When it happens, the gene creates proteins that can cause cancer to grow and spread. This is seen in some lung, colon, soft tissue, head and neck, thyroid, and brain cancers.

PD-L1: PD-L1 (programmed cell death ligand 1) is a protein that plays a role in the body's immune system. It can bind to another protein called PD-1. When this happens, the two proteins block the immune system from killing cancer cells. Doctors have figured out how to prevent the two proteins from binding and help the immune system do its job in removing cancer cells.

RET: RET proto-oncogene is a gene that plays a role in cell signaling. The *RET* gene can change and join with other genes. This is called *RET* fusion. When it happens, cancer can grow and spread.

ROS1: ROS1 is the gene that makes the protein ROS1. It plays a role in cell signaling and cell growth. A change in ROS1 or too much ROS1 can cause cancer to grow and spread. This is seen in some lung, colorectal, stomach, ovarian, bile duct, and brain cancers.

When you have cancer, it is important to talk with your doctor about biomarker testing. Ask if there are biomarker tests indicated for your type and stage of cancer. Ask how they might inform the treatment plan. Biomarker testing can be hard to understand, so be sure to ask questions and ask again if you don't understand. Use the resources listed here to learn more about genetic and genomic testing.

RESOURCES TO LEARN MORE ABOUT GENETICS AND GENETIC TESTING

Cancer Support Community's "Is Cancer Hereditary?"—Learn more about inherited cancer syndromes and when and how to get tested. www.cancersupportcommunity.org/cancer-hereditary

National Cancer Institute's "The Genetics of Cancer"—www.cancer.gov/about-cancer/causes-prevention/genetics

National Society of Genetic Counselors—Learn more about genetic testing and find a genetic counselor in your community. www.nsgc.org

RESOURCES TO LEARN MORE ABOUT GENOMICS AND BIOMARKER TESTING

Cancer Support Community's "Precision Medicine"—Learn more about biomarkers and targeted therapy through written content and videos. www.cancersupportcommunity.org/article/precision-medicine

"Mutations Matter"—Learn more about biomarker testing from this brief video put out by the Cholangiocarcinoma Foundation. www.youtube.com/watch?v=XOiJK_rMKuM

National Cancer Institute's "Cancer Genomics Overview"—Includes more background on targeted therapy and its role in cancer treatment. www.cancer.gov/about-nci/organization/ccg/cancer-genomics-overview

The resources above relate to all biomarkers. If you have tested positive for a specific biomarker, you may be able to find an online source of information and support for people with that biomarker. Examples include: www.egfrcancer.org, alkpositive.org, ros1cancer.com, and exon20group.org.

CHAPTER 6

Make an Informed Treatment Decision

You now have a complete diagnosis, including all necessary tests and scans, and you've learned what it means. The next step is to decide on a treatment plan. You and your health care team will work together to come up with the right plan for you. Your treatment plan should take into account your treatment goals and priorities. You and your team will consider your lifestyle, support network, and what makes the most sense for you at this time.

In some instances, the treatment plan for your cancer may be clear. Your doctor will recommend a course of action based on their opinion and experience, and the treatment guidelines we reviewed in chapter four. In other cases, you may have options for treatment. Your doctor may ask you to weigh in on your preference. For example, in early-stage breast cancer, your doctor may ask you to choose between a lumpectomy and a mastectomy. You have a choice because doctors have found that these two approaches have similar clinical outcomes for the type of cancer you have. Or your doctor may offer you a standard treatment or the option to participate in a clinical trial. (We will cover the basics of clinical trials in chapter eight.)

As cancer diagnosis and treatment have become more complex, patients are more often asked to make choices. Sometimes this can feel overwhelming. If you are in this situation, you may choose to let your doctor make the decision—which is perfectly fine. Or you may want to be more involved in the decision-making but aren't sure how to do that.

In health care today, we often talk about shared decision-making. This means engaging in a dialogue with your doctor and your team. You talk through all aspects of your care and jointly arrive at a decision. Your doctor will present the treatment options and describe possible outcomes, side effects, and other factors to consider. Even with this information, it may be hard to make a decision that feels right for you. Let's review some different ways to think about treatment and put the decision in the context of your life and values. **Remember, there isn't a right decision; there is only a decision that is right for you.**

"Don't be afraid to talk to your doctor about what you like. If you want all the information, then make sure you get it. If you don't really want to know everything, then make sure that's clear too. And sometimes we don't know what we want but as you go along, don't be afraid to ask for what you need."
—Mariann, breast cancer survivor and former caregiver

First, as we mentioned earlier, it is important to know as much about your cancer and the possible treatments as possible. Consider these questions to get started:

- What type and subtype of cancer do you have?
- What is the stage or grade of disease?
- How and where will the treatment be given? For how many weeks or months? How often?
- Does this treatment plan follow the standard of care or national guidelines?
- What are the possible side effects, and how do you prepare for those?

Next, think about your lifestyle and the support network around you:

- Do you live alone or with other people?
- Do you work? Can your work be done from home?
- Do you have a caregiver in the home, or at a distance?
- Do you have any disabilities or other health conditions that need to be considered?
- Do you have concerns about your home? Are there stairs to contend with? Do you have easy access to a bathroom?
- Will you have challenges getting back and forth to treatment?

Consider your short- and long-term goals:

- Are you hoping to be well enough to attend a child or grandchild's graduation? Take a trip you have planned? Attend a family wedding?
- Do you want to be able to walk your dog or cook a meal for your family or yourself?

These are all important things to discuss with your health care team so they can get to know you as a person and tailor a treatment plan for you. Ask your team how much time you have to make a decision. Seek support in the decision-making process.

---

*"When it was time for treatment, my doctor gave me some options.
I think there were three of them. Along with my children, we decided right then and there at the visit what was best for me, and the oncologist agreed as well, so it ended up being an oral medication with fewer side effects."*
—Lynn, chronic lymphocytic leukemia survivor

TIPS FOR TREATMENT PLANNING[1]

Listen to answers. Any questions you have about the cancer and its treatment are worth asking. Listen closely and keep asking questions until you understand what is being said. Ask for information in a different language or format (like a drawing) if you need to. *Bring a friend or relative to take notes or record the doctor,* if the doctor is okay with that.

Think about the pros and cons. Your family, friends, current patients, and your health care team can help you think through your options before you pick a path. Ask how likely it is for each treatment path to work for you.

Ask about side effects. What side effects should you expect for each treatment type? When do they usually start? How long do they last? How do you manage them?

Ask about costs. Is this treatment covered by your insurance? If not, can you get help paying for it? Are there programs that can help you with other costs (prescriptions, childcare, household costs) while you are in treatment?

Ask about your time commitment. How often will you need to go to the clinic? How long will you be there? How much work will you miss? Will you need help with child or elder care?

Ask about travel. Where will you go for treatment? How will you get there? Is transportation assistance an option?

---

1. Cancer Support Community, *Frankly Speaking About Cancer: Multiple Myeloma,* February 2019, www.cancersupportcommunity.org/multiple-myeloma.

At the Cancer Support Community, we have a model of treatment-decision counseling called Open to Options. Open to Options is a structured session with a trained specialist who helps a patient, in a nondirective way, develop a question list centered on the patient's own values, preferences, and priorities. It can take place in person or by phone. The patient can then take the list back to the doctor to discuss treatment options and next steps. Below is an example of an Open to Options list developed by the Cancer Support Community's clinical team that could come out of a session with a counselor. This is only an example and is not based on an actual patient.

SITUATION (known facts about my condition)

I was originally diagnosed with breast cancer in 2013.

It spread to my bones in 2015.

I was on treatment until my cancer spread to my pyloric sphincter.

I now have a feeding tube.

I have recently been taken off chemotherapy because of blistering on my feet.

OPTIONS (possible treatment options)

More chemotherapy was mentioned.

I've heard about clinical trials, but I don't know a lot.

I have a second opinion next week about possible options.

NETWORK (personal and medical)

My current oncologist is Dr. Y.

Dr. S. is my family doctor. I have seen her for over twenty years and I trust her.

Nurse Diane is my chemo nurse. She has been a real support.

My husband, Jim, has some memory issues.

My two adult children live out of state.

My Cancer Support Community support group is so supportive.

I have many neighbors who help with transportation and yard work.

GOALS (my goals and priorities)

I want to be able to eat.

If I need more chemo, I want to be back to normal as soon as possible.

My daughter is getting married in six months and I want to attend the wedding, which is out of state.

Walking for exercise is very important to me.

I need to take care of my husband.

I want to have the same quality of life that I had with palbociclib.

EVALUATION (how my options may affect my goals)

Is there a treatment that will be more or less likely to cause chemo brain?

Is a clinical trial an option for me?

Is there a treatment that could cure me?

If I can't be cured, which treatment will give me more time and the best quality of life?

Is removing the feeding tube a possibility?

If I need more chemotherapy, is there one with the same side effects as the chemotherapy I was on before?

Can I travel to my daughter's wedding?

Taking the time to plan and talk with your health care team will allow you to be more informed and empowered as you face the weeks and months ahead. It will also ensure that your own values, preferences, and priorities are factored into the overall care plan.

RESOURCES FOR TREATMENT PLANNING

Cancer Support Community's *Frankly Speaking About Cancer: Making Treatment Decisions*—A must-read for patients on the verge of making treatment decisions. www.CancerSupportCommunity.org/sites/default/files/fsac/Making_Treatment _DecisionsBooklet.pdf

Cancer Support Community's "Making a Treatment Decision That Is Right for You"— Resources and support to help make treatment decisions, including links to the CSC's decision support counseling program, Open to Options. www.cancersupport community.org/OpentoOptions

CHAPTER 7

Get a Second Opinion

It is common for people with cancer to seek a second opinion. A second opinion is just what it sounds like. It's what you get when you go to a second doctor for further input. This doctor is usually at a different hospital or cancer center. You ask their opinion of your diagnosis and the recommended treatment. People with cancer often go to a large academic medical center or a National Cancer Institute (NCI)–designated comprehensive cancer center for a second opinion.

"It's important to get two opinions because different institutions do different things. You need to check out your options and decide what you are comfortable with."
—Laura, multiple myeloma survivor

WHAT IS AN NCI-DESIGNATED COMPREHENSIVE CANCER CENTER, AND WHY IS IT IMPORTANT?

NCI cancer centers are hospitals and cancer centers that receive funding from the U.S. government for excellence in cancer research and treatment. They are part of the NCI Cancer Centers Program. According to the NCI, the Cancer Centers Program "was created as part of the National Cancer Act of 1971 and is one of the anchors of the nation's cancer research effort. Through this program, NCI recognizes centers around the country that meet rigorous standards for transdisciplinary, state-of-the-art research focused on developing new and better approaches to preventing, diagnosing, and treating cancer."[1] The seventy-one cancer centers are in thirty-six states and the District of Columbia. Being an NCI cancer center is an honor. Hospitals work hard to get on this list and stay on it. These centers often have the latest cancer treatments and clinical trials.

---

1. "NCI-Designated Cancer Centers," National Cancer Institute, accessed November 13, 2020, www.cancer.gov/research/nci-role/cancer-centers.

Patients choose to seek a second, or even a third, opinion for a host of different reasons. Let's go over some here:

- A second opinion, especially at a large academic center, may reveal more treatment options that make sense for you. The appointment is often with an expert in the field or a doctor who has a lot of experience in treating the specific cancer you have.

- A second opinion means, of course, that you have seen a first doctor. You may want to explore other options or hear a different point of view. Treating cancer is both an art and a science. Your health care team will consult the treatment guidelines we discussed in chapter four and talk with colleagues. They will look at current research and rely on their clinical experience and judgment. Different doctors take different approaches, so it might be helpful to hear from more than one as you think about the path forward.

- When you have cancer, it is likely that you will spend a lot of time at the hospital or clinic where you are being treated and with your health care team. It is important, therefore, that you like them and that they treat you with dignity and respect. You need to feel comfortable and confident in their care. Some people seek a second opinion to look for a team or hospital that feels like a better fit.

- A second opinion may lead you to a clinical trial that might be right for you. A clinical trial is a study that tests a new treatment or a new way to use an existing treatment. Every drug that is used today has been tested in clinical trials. This means that it went through a rigorous approval process before becoming available. On a cancer treatment trial, you will likely receive either the standard of care—the recommended treatment for your kind of cancer—or the standard of care plus the new drug that is being studied. In either case, you will receive treatment for cancer. We will talk more about clinical trials in the next chapter.

You may worry that getting a second opinion will interfere with your cancer treatment goals. You may be thinking:

- *I don't have time to get a second opinion. I want to get started with treatment right away.* If this concerns you, ask the first doctor you saw how much time you have to make a decision. Your doctor may say that the cancer is aggressive and they want to start treatment right away. Or your doctor may say you have some time to decide how you would like to proceed. In most cases, you will have time to seek a second opinion and weigh your options.

- *I can't afford a second opinion.* In general, Medicare, Medicaid, and most private insurers will pay for a second opinion when you have cancer. Each plan (and provider network) is different, so it is a good idea to call your plan to ask. We will talk more about insurance in chapter nine.

- *I don't want to upset or offend my doctor. I don't want my doctor to see me as a "difficult" patient. I don't want to "rock the boat."* In general, a doctor who treats cancer will find it normal and acceptable for you to seek a second opinion. Some even suggest it. A doctor who is offended that you would seek a second opinion may not be the right doctor for you.

"My doctor encouraged me to get a second opinion. He told me to get two or three.
It was very reassuring to know that he had my best interests in mind."
—Amanda, metastatic breast cancer survivor

Lastly, as you prepare for your second opinion visit, gather all your records and scans from the first doctor. The second doctor will need these to provide an opinion. Try to obtain your records electronically and send them in advance. If that is not possible, ask for hard copies and bring them with you to the second opinion appointment. Your records may include biopsy and pathology reports, images from scans (e.g., CT scans, PET scans, or X-rays), the results of blood work, or the findings from genetic or bio-marker tests. Also bring a list of any medicines you are taking and their doses. Having this information ready will help the visit go more smoothly and quickly.

THE BENEFITS OF A SECOND OPINION[2]

- To confirm your diagnosis
- To get more information about your treatment now and in the future
- To learn about possible clinical trials
- To help you choose the doctor and treatment team you want to work with
- To learn about different treatment locations (e.g., a community clinic, a local hospital, an academic medical center, or an NCI-designated cancer center)
- To learn about what services each treatment location can offer
- To make sure that your insurance company will pay for your cancer treatment (some companies require a second opinion)

---

2. Cancer Support Community, *Frankly Speaking About Cancer: Multiple Myeloma,* February 2019, www.cancersupportcommunity.org/multiple-myeloma.

———————————

"Hearing from so many other women was very helpful. I wanted to stay in my little cocoon of my original decision, and then my good friend, you know, she kind of begged me to listen to other people, and to just go for a second opinion in Philadelphia, and I was very, very grateful for that."
—Lisa, breast cancer survivor

———————————

RESOURCES FOR FINDING A HOSPITAL OR DOCTOR

American College of Surgeons—Find a surgeon or accredited cancer program. www.facs
.org/search/cancer-programs

American Society of Clinical Oncology—Find a cancer doctor on the website of the
world's largest professional organization for medical oncologists. www.cancer.net
/find-cancer doctor

National Cancer Institute (NCI)—Find a multidisciplinary care team at an NCI-
designated comprehensive cancer center, a hospital, or cancer center in the United
States recognized for leading cancer research and care. www.cancer.gov/research/nci
-role/cancer-centers/find

CHAPTER 8

Ask About Clinical Trials

Clinical trials are medical research studies with patients. Cancer trials test whether new drugs or other treatments are safe and effective for the prevention, diagnosis, or treatment of cancer. The drugs in clinical trials were studied in labs for many years before being studied in people. Any drug that is on the market today went through an extremely rigorous research approval process. This process has many steps that often span years. The Food and Drug Administration (FDA) is the government agency that regulates drugs in the United States. It also oversees the safety of food, cosmetics, medical devices, medications for animals, and more. The FDA must approve a drug before it is sold to people. This is true for both prescription and over-the-counter drugs.

Before you say, "I don't want to be in a clinical trial," and skip this chapter, let's go over some myths and facts about clinical trials. Then we will talk about how to find and join a trial and why you might want to consider one. We will also touch on key words to know, including the different phases of trials and what they mean.

"We were given a lot of information before I decided to join. There was absolutely no pressure to sign on the dotted line the day that I found out about the study."
—Mary Clare, acute myeloid leukemia survivor

MYTHS AND FACTS ABOUT CLINICAL TRIALS

MYTH: All clinical trials have a placebo. A placebo is a harmless pill or medicine that has no therapeutic effect or value. It is sometimes called a sugar pill.

FACT: Almost no cancer treatment trials contain a placebo. It would be unethical to deny a cancer patient, at minimum, standard therapy for their cancer. If you are in a cancer treatment trial, you will, in all likelihood, get treatment.

MYTH: You should consider a clinical trial only as a last-ditch effort when all other treatments have failed.

FACT: In general, there are clinical trials for many different cancers at various stages of disease. Ask your doctor if there might be a trial that is right for you.

MYTH: I will be treated like a guinea pig or a lab rat if I participate in a trial.

FACT: Studies show that a significant percentage of patients who participate in trials have a very positive experience. In most trials, you will be monitored very closely. You will have regular visits to the office for check-ins, scans, blood work, and other care. There are no "guinea pigs" or "lab rats" in cancer clinical trials. A drug has to go through extensive safety testing and reviews before being offered in a clinical trial.

MYTH: It is expensive to participate in a trial.

FACT: The costs of the trial and trial drugs are generally covered by health insurance and the drug manufacturer. They might even include a stipend to help with added costs like parking and gas. If you have concerns about extra costs (like childcare or hotels), tell the clinical trial coordinator. There may be additional resources to help.

HOW DO I FIND A CLINICAL TRIAL?

If you are trying to find a clinical trial, the first step is to talk with your doctor. Ask if there are any clinical trials at your hospital or clinic or in your local area that you should consider. Also ask about trials in other parts of the country.

Your doctor may or may not be aware of trials. If they do not know of any, ask if someone on the team can help you look for possible trials. You or a family member can also search for trials in the federal government database at www.clinicaltrials.gov. This site is run by the U.S. National Library of Medicine at the National Institutes of Health. It is said to be the largest clinical trials database in the world. Because of this, the information may not be completely up-to-date. If you find a trial in the database that is of interest to you, discuss it with your doctor. Every clinical trial has eligibility criteria. Your doctor can tell you if you might qualify. Also, contact the trial site to see if the trial is still open and enrolling patients.

"By the grace of God, I'm still here because of clinical trials. They are scary and you don't know what will or will not happen because the treatments are new. But if you are willing to take that chance, those are options. You need to educate yourself, advocate for yourself, and get second opinions."

—Kristen, acute lymphoblastic leukemia survivor

HOW DO I JOIN A CLINICAL TRIAL?

Before joining a clinical trial, you will be asked to sign a document called an informed consent. This document is usually long and sometimes complicated. It outlines all the details of the trial, including the goals and possible risks and benefits. By signing it, you agree to participate; however, you are free to withdraw from a clinical trial at any point and for any reason. It is important that you go over this document carefully with your doctor or the clinical trial coordinator. A clinical trial coordinator is a person who organizes all aspects of the trial. This person will become your primary contact while you are in the trial.

As you consider participating in a trial, ask as many questions as you'd like; don't hesitate to ask again if you do not understand something. Be sure to include your caregiver or trusted friend in the conversation too. Some questions to ask include:[1]

- *What is the goal of this trial?* Before you sign, get clarity on what the trial is studying. For example, ask: Is the goal of the trial to cure my cancer? To help me live longer than if I was on standard treatment? Is it to slow the growth of the cancer? These questions will help you decide whether you want to participate.
- *What are the risks and benefits of the new treatment?* This is a good time to ask about possible side effects.
- *How does the treatment on this trial compare to the other treatments I am considering?* A trial is one of your treatment options. Be sure to ask all the same questions that you would ask about any treatment you consider.
- *What will I have to do as a participant in this trial?* Ask how often you will be expected to visit the hospital or clinic. What kind of tests will the doctors do? Will they check in with you in other ways, such as phone calls?
- *How long will I be on this trial?* The trial could take months or years. Some trials have an end date. The end date may depend on how well the treatment is working.
- *Is this trial covered by my insurance?* What will I have to pay out of pocket?

The answers to these questions will help you decide if this clinical trial is right for you.

---

1. Cancer Support Community, *Frankly Speaking About Cancer: Coping with Side Effects*, December 2019, www.cancersupportcommunity.org/sites/default/files/fields/resource/file/2020 -01/coping_with_side_effects_book.pdf.

THE LANGUAGE OF CLINICAL TRIALS[2]

As you learn about clinical trials, you may hear some words that are not familiar to you. Let's go over some definitions, starting with the phases of trials. Every clinical trial has a phase, as follows:

Preclinical trial: Drugs are studied in labs, usually in animals, for years before they are tested on people. Only drugs that have a scientific basis and show the promise of benefit make it past this phase.

Phase I: Once a drug is approved and determined safe for human studies, it is tested in a small trial to determine the optimal best dose. These studies monitor patients very closely for side effects. Phase I studies often involve patients with different kinds of cancer.

Phase II: If a drug can be given safely to people in the phase I trial, it is tested in a phase II study. These are larger studies, usually for one or more specific types and stages of cancer. The goal of phase II studies is both to determine the optimal dosing and to provide an early assessment of whether the drug works.

Phase III: These trials take place after a drug has shown good results in earlier studies. They are large studies. They often involve hundreds or even thousands of patients, in different hospitals in the United States and/or abroad. Patients in phase III trials have specific types and stages of cancer. Many phase III trials are randomized. This means that patients are randomly assigned to receive either the new treatment or the standard of care. These trials are designed to provide evidence to support FDA approval of the drug for use in the public.

Phase IV: These trials take place after a drug is approved and are often called postmarketing trials. The goal is to make sure that no safety or

---

2. Adapted from "Clinical Trials for Cancer," Cancer Support Community, accessed November 17, 2020, www.cancersupportcommunity.org/clinical-trials-cancer.

other concerns have come up since approval. It is important to follow patients for many years to determine if there are any long-term side effects or other issues that affect the way the treatment is used.

These key terms refer to how trials are structured:[3]

Blinded: A type of study in which the patients do not know which drug or treatment is being given. This is also called single-blinded. The opposite of a blinded study is an open-label study.

Double-blinded: A type of study in which both the patients and their doctors do not know which drug or treatment is being given to which patients.

Randomized: A study in which the participants are divided by chance into separate groups to compare different treatments. Using chance to divide people into groups means that the groups will be similar. The effects of the treatments they receive can be compared more fairly. At the time of the trial, it is not known which treatment is best.

Inclusion and exclusion criteria: The characteristics that make patients eligible or ineligible for a clinical trial. They can relate to the type and stage of cancer or to the presence of certain biomarkers. Patients also may be included or excluded based on the treatments they have already tried and their responses to them.

---

3. NCI Dictionary of Cancer Terms, National Cancer Institute, accessed October 19, 2020, www.cancer.gov/publications/dictionaries/cancer-terms.

Clinical trials are an important part of cancer treatment. Sometimes, the newest and most promising treatment is available only through a trial. You may join because you see it as the best hope for recovery. Some people join a clinical trial because they want the opportunity to be part of science or to help others. We hear patients say, "I don't know if I will benefit from this treatment in my lifetime, but perhaps someone else will benefit in the future."

Such altruistic motives are inspiring and give us faith in humanity and people's commitment to the greater good. Whatever you ultimately decide, it is a good idea to ask about a clinical trial as a possible treatment option and explore whether a trial might be right for you.

"When I was first diagnosed with prostate cancer, it was a total surprise. I was devastated. I did a whole lot of research; I interviewed with five different doctors at three major teaching hospitals before I decided on one. It turned out to be the hospital where a doctor was offering a clinical trial and he was very encouraging to go into the trial."
—Glen, prostate cancer and Merkel cell carcinoma survivor

Clinical Trials

HOLLY ROWE

Holly Rowe is one of ESPN's most versatile commentators and an Emmy-nominated reporter. Since her cancer diagnosis, Rowe has become an unwavering advocate for cancer research and prevention.

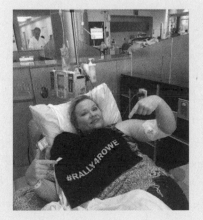

*C*linical trial used to be a phrase I only ever heard in those feel-good pharmaceutical commercials on TV. I didn't know how a clinical trial would dramatically impact my life negatively and then positively one day.

I was diagnosed with stage 3c melanoma in 2015. At that time, the lifesaving treatments for immunotherapy had not been FDA approved for my stage of cancer. As crazy as it may sound, I was wishing my diagnosis was stage 4 so I could be eligible for the new melanoma treatments that I was reading were very successful. Instead, I was offered a clinical trial in which I would be randomized into a treatment protocol. Basically, a computer would choose if I could get immunotherapy or a traditional melanoma cancer drug called interferon.

I was randomized to high-dose interferon. I went through nearly a month of high-dose treatments that ravaged me. I was so sick I couldn't function. I really struggled. After all that, the melanoma spread anyway.

With new tumors in my lungs, I was now a candidate for immunotherapy. I changed doctors and went to the UCLA medical center where Dr. Toni Ribas, one of the top melanoma researchers in the country, taught me about a clinical trial that was available. I truly believe being in a clinical trial helped save me. The tumors in my lungs are no longer visible.

It was crucial for me to be a part of a clinical trial to get access to treatment that was not FDA approved for my stage of cancer at that time. Also, it helped alleviate the financial impact. Immunotherapy at that time was very expensive and being in the clinical trial saved me and my insurance company potentially hundreds of thousands of dollars. I also felt the importance of furthering research and helping others with my same diagnosis. I am so grateful to have had the opportunity to be in a trial.

When you are diagnosed with cancer, it can be overwhelming, but I truly believe one of the *first* questions you should ask is, "Am I a candidate for a clinical trial?"

RESOURCES TO LEARN MORE ABOUT CLINICAL TRIALS

Cancer Support Community's "Cancer Clinical Trials"—Learn more about clinical trials and use the Cancer Support Community's matching service to find a trial that might be right for you. www.CancerSupportCommunity.org/clinical-trials-cancer

National Cancer Institute's Clinical Trials Registry—This phone line or website lets you answer five questions and get a list of trials that might be right for you. 800-422-6237 or www.cancer.gov/clinicaltrials

National Library of Medicine's Clinical Trials Search—This is a searchable database of publicly and privately funded clinical trials being conducted around the world. www.clinicaltrials.gov

CHAPTER 9

Get to Know Your Insurance Coverage

It will come as no surprise that cancer treatment is costly. In the United States, health insurance is essential. But it can also be confusing, and not all insurance plans are the same. And not everyone has insurance. Whether you have insurance or not, this chapter is for you.

IF YOU HAVE INSURANCE

It is often said that you don't know how good (or bad!) your health insurance is until you face a serious illness. One of the first things you want to do is find out what your insurance covers. Most of us don't know the ins and outs of our insurance policies. We might not even be able to easily put our hands on a copy! Now is the time to dust off that policy. If you can't find it and are employed, ask the human resources person at work for one. Your insurance company should also be able to provide a copy. This is also a good time to find out if your hospital has a financial counselor on staff. This person may be able to help answer your insurance questions.

IF YOU DON'T HAVE INSURANCE

If you don't have insurance, you may be feeling a little panicked. Start by taking a deep breath. We can help. Step one is to use your resources to see if you might be able to obtain insurance. Start with your health care team. Ask if your hospital or clinic has a social worker or financial counselor on staff. If so, find out the best way to reach them. Try to begin the paperwork right away, before the bills pile up. Your health care team also may be able to refer you to a community or nonprofit organization that can help. The process will take some time, but you may be able to get insurance. If you are having trouble getting answers to your questions, call the Cancer Support Helpline at 888-793-9355.

When you start looking into insurance, you may hear some new words. Knowing these words will help you talk with billing offices and your insurance company. Let's begin by reviewing the different kinds of coverage that are out there:[1]

Private insurance: Private insurance comes from a company. You may get it through work or a union or buy it directly from the company. Insurance that is not private comes from the government.

Medicare: This is a federal health insurance program for people ages sixty-five and older and certain younger people with disabilities. It is sometimes called "Original Medicare." It has two parts—A and B.

Medicare Advantage (Medicare Part C): With this plan, you receive coverage through a private company. The company contracts with Medicare to provide your benefits. You are covered for the services included in Original Medicare, and some extras. You also may be able to choose the type of plan you have (read on for more on types of plans). If you have questions about your coverage, call the company.

Medicare Part D: This program helps pay for prescription drugs for people with Medicare who join a plan that includes prescription drug coverage. There are two ways to get Medicare prescription drug coverage: through a Medicare Prescription Drug Plan or a Medicare Advantage Plan that includes drug coverage. These plans are offered by insurance companies and other private companies approved by Medicare.

---

1. Definitions from or adapted from HealthCare.gov Glossary, accessed October 20, 2020, www .healthcare.gov/glossary.

Medicaid: This program provides free or low-cost health coverage to some low-income people, families and children, pregnant women, elderly people, and people with disabilities. Many states have expanded Medicaid to cover all people below certain income levels. Whether you qualify for Medicaid depends partly on whether your state has expanded its program. Medicaid benefits and program names vary by state. You can apply anytime. If you qualify, your coverage can begin right away, at any time of year.

TRICARE: This is a health care program for active-duty and retired uniformed services members and their families.

If you have private insurance or Medicare Part C, you might have a choice of what kind of insurance plan you buy. Major types include:[2]

Health maintenance organization (HMO): A plan in which you choose from a network of doctors in one area. It generally won't cover out-of-network care except in an emergency. There is often a focus on prevention and wellness.

Point-of-service plan (POS): A plan in which you pay less if you use doctors, hospitals, and other health care providers that belong to the plan's network. POS plans require you to get a referral from your primary care doctor in order to see a specialist.

Preferred provider organization (PPO): A plan that contracts with hospitals and doctors to create a network of providers. You pay less if you use providers that belong to the plan's network. You can use doctors, hospitals, and providers outside the network for an added cost.

Health savings account (HSA): A type of savings account that lets you set aside money on a pretax basis to pay for some medical costs. By using untaxed dollars in an HSA, you may be able to lower your health care costs. HSA funds generally may not be used to pay premiums.

High-deductible health plan (HDHP): A plan with a higher deductible than a traditional insurance plan. The monthly premium is usually lower, but you pay more before the insurance company starts to pay its share. An HDHP can be combined

---

2. Definitions from or adapted from the glossary found at HealthCare.gov.

with an HSA. This may allow you to pay for certain medical expenses with money free from federal taxes.

As discussed, most people get health insurance through work, Medicare, Medicaid, or the military. However, some people buy their insurance on what is called the state health insurance marketplace or exchange. The marketplaces were put in place in 2010 after the U.S. Congress passed the Patient Protection and Affordable Care Act, also known as the ACA (or, informally, Obamacare). They allow people without insurance (who are not eligible for Medicare) to buy private health insurance through the state where they live. To learn more about the state exchanges, you can visit HealthCare.gov.

Regardless of the type of insurance you have, here are some common terms you may encounter when reviewing your policy:[3]

Premium: The amount you and/or your employer pay each month for the insurance coverage.

Co-payment (co-pay): The amount your insurance requires you to pay each time you receive care.

Deductible: The amount of approved health care costs you must pay out of pocket each year before your insurance begins paying any costs.

Coinsurance: The percentage of costs you pay after meeting your health care plan's annual deductible.

Specialty pharmacies: Some pharmacies offer added services and resources for patients with cancer or other chronic illnesses. They may use mail order. Doctors order drugs through them to get lower co-pays for patients.

Explanation of benefits (EOB): A document that outlines what portion of your health care charges will be paid by your insurance plan.

Out-of-pocket maximum: The most you must pay for covered services in a plan year. After you spend this amount on deductibles, co-pays, and coinsurance, your health plan pays 100 percent of the costs of covered benefits.

---

3. Definitions from or adapted from the glossary found at HealthCare.gov.

COBRA: This federal law allows you to keep your insurance for a certain amount of time after your job ends. You will have to pay more for this coverage than you paid through work.

Even when you have insurance, you may face problems. Patients sometimes tell us that their insurance provider has denied coverage for a test, procedure, or drug. This can be upsetting and frustrating. Know that you can try to appeal the company's decision. If you are in this situation, start by asking your doctor's office for help. If the denial is for a specific drug, the company that makes it may have case managers or financial counselors who can help with the appeal process. There are also community and advocacy organizations that can help with an appeal.

TIPS FOR THE APPEALS PROCESS[4]

- Make sure you have a copy of the denial letter. If you don't already have a copy, ask the insurance company to send you one.
- Make note of the deadline by which you must submit an appeal for it to be considered.
- The denial letter must document the specific reason that the claim or pre-authorization was denied.
- Get a copy of your current insurance benefit plan. This may be available online, or you may have to request a copy of it in writing.
- If you receive health insurance through your employer and you are comfortable sharing information about your medical condition with them, consider asking for help communicating with the insurance company.

(continued)

_____

4. "Tips for Appealing a Denial of Coverage," Cancer Support Community, accessed November 13, 2020, www.cancersupportcommunity.org/coping-cost -care/health-insurance-cancer-patients.

- Consider asking a family member or a friend to "quarterback" or take the lead and help manage the appeal and other paperwork, which can lessen the stress of an appeals process.
- Ask what you need to do to request a "doctor-to-doctor" conversation. This is a process by which your doctor can talk directly to the medical director at the health insurance company.
- As you go through the appeals process, take careful notes. Write down the names and direct phone numbers of people you speak with, when (date and time), and the nature of the call.
- Be certain to try all external appeals that are available in your state.
- Hang in there. Appeals take persistence. Careful note-taking will allow you to hand off the process to someone who is helping you if you want to take a break from all the phone calls.

We also hear from patients that sometimes the co-pays on their drugs are well beyond what they can afford. A number of foundations and nonprofit organizations provide what is called co-pay assistance. Some are listed below. Contact these groups to see if they can help. Also, as we mentioned earlier, the pharmaceutical company that makes the drug may have assistance available. Be sure to reach out to them as well.

Organizations that provide co-pay assistance:

- CancerCare—www.cancercare.org
- Cancer Financial Assistance Coalition—www.cancerfac.org
- HealthWell Foundation—www.healthwellfoundation.org
- Leukemia and Lymphoma Society Co-Pay Assistance Program—www.lls.org /support/financial-support/co-pay-assistance-program
- Patient Advocate Foundation Co-Pay Relief Fund—www.patientadvocate.org /connect-with-services/copay-relief/
- Patient Access Network (PAN) Foundation—www.panfoundation.org

There are many more organizations than we can list here. The important takeaway is that help is out there. Don't be afraid to ask and use the resources in the back of this book.

"I have been very fortunate to have good insurance. With the amount of surgeries and treatments that I've had over time, I've gotten good at playing this insurance game. I know how much my insurance is going to pay. Yes, I've had to call the hospital at times to find out how much an MRI or scan is going to cost. I know my insurance is going to pay 90 percent of it so I calculate what my 10 percent is going to be. Even with them paying so much, my co-pays, premiums, and the 10 percent all add up. It gets expensive."

—Christy, head and neck cancer survivor

RESOURCES TO LEARN MORE ABOUT HEALTH INSURANCE

Cancer Support Community's "Managing the Cost of Cancer Treatment"—Links to many helpful resources, including the following two essential publications on the topic. www.cancersupportcommunity.org/managing-cost-cancer-treatment

- Cancer Support Community's *Frankly Speaking About Cancer: Tips for Managing and Budgeting Your Cancer Costs*
- Cancer Support Community's book *Frankly Speaking About Cancer: Coping with the Cost of Care*

HealthCare.gov—Research the insurance marketplace options in your state. www.healthcare.gov

Medicare—Look up public insurance options for adults sixty-five and older. www.medicare.gov

Patient Access Network (PAN) Foundation—Helps with out-of-pocket medical costs. www.panfoundation.org

Patient Advocate Foundation—Provides advocacy and support to patients. www.patientadvocate.org

Triage Cancer—Learn more about the legal and financial side of coping with cancer. triagecancer.org

CHAPTER 10

Ask to Be Screened for Distress

We have talked quite a bit in the early chapters of this book about the tools used to diagnose and treat cancer. But there is another tool that is just as important. That tool is a screening that is vital to your health and well-being—screening for distress.

What does screening for distress mean? It is very common when facing a cancer diagnosis to be scared, anxious, depressed, or worried about a wide range of issues. This may include practical matters like money, your job, your family, or the logistics of care. Or you might find yourself thinking about your own mortality. This is all normal, but it's also normal to need and get help coping with cancer. Screening for distress is like a check-in. Your health care team should ask you how you are doing and be ready to connect you to resources to address any concerns.

BACKGROUND

It seems obvious that doctors should care about the mental well-being of people with cancer. But, in fact, it is a somewhat new idea. In 2008, the National Academy of Medicine (then called the Institute of Medicine) issued a report called "Cancer Care for the Whole Patient: Meeting Psychosocial Health Needs." The report stressed the need to take care of the whole person, not just treat cancer.

Not long after that report was issued, the Commission on Cancer (CoC) of the American College of Surgeons took a bold step. This body, which accredits cancer programs across the United States, added distress screening to its review process. This means that the CoC now looks at how a hospital or cancer center meets the nonmedical needs of patients. This factor is considered alongside medical concerns, like how well they administer chemo and manage pain, as examples. The CoC wants cancer programs to ask patients about distress and connect them to help both inside and outside the hospital.

WHAT THIS MEANS FOR YOU

So, what does screening for distress look like? How does it work? In general, it works like a survey. It usually takes place at the beginning of a doctor's visit or while you are waiting in the exam room. You may be given a computer or tablet, or possibly pen and paper. The survey will include questions about how you are feeling. It will ask how concerned you are about different aspects of your health and life. Based on your answers, the team will sit down with you to go through your responses. If needed, they will connect you with resources that can help. In a hospital or clinic, this process is likely to be led by a psychologist, a social worker, a nurse navigator, or a case manager. If you do not receive a survey like this, be sure to ask for one.

There are many screening tools out there. Each hospital may use a different one. At the Cancer Support Community, we screen the patients and caregivers who visit our fifty affiliate locations across North America. We use our own fifteen-item, scientifically validated screening tool called Cancer Support Source. Patients take the screener on a tablet, then sit with a social worker to review the results and create a customized care plan.

Here are a few examples of questions in the Cancer Support Source screener. Each includes a follow-up question about how the Cancer Support Community can help.

Today, how concerned are you about sleep problems? (Please circle one option)

1	2	3	4	5
Not at all	Slightly	Moderately	Seriously	Very Seriously

Please let us know how we can help you:
- ❏ Have a staff person talk with you
- ❏ Provide you additional information
- ❏ No action needed

Today, how concerned are you about health insurance or money worries? (Please circle one option)

1	2	3	4	5
Not at all	Slightly	Moderately	Seriously	Very Seriously

Please let us know how we can help you:
- ❏ Have a staff person talk with you
- ❏ Provide you additional information
- ❏ No action needed

Today, how concerned are you about feeling lonely or isolated? (Please circle one option)

1	2	3	4	5
Not at all	Slightly	Moderately	Seriously	Very Seriously

Please let us know how we can help you:
- ❏ Have a staff person talk with you
- ❏ Provide you additional information
- ❏ No action needed

These simple questions offer a way to help people beyond chemo, radiation, or other medical treatment. Screening patients for distress is not just about social and emotional health. Stress can weaken our immune systems,[1] which may affect the body's ability to fight cancer.

By addressing patients' practical, social, emotional, financial, and spiritual needs, we are treating the whole person, not just the disease. We are able to remove barriers to care and help build a support network and a complete care team, paving the way for the best possible outcomes.

RESOURCES TO LEARN MORE ABOUT SCREENING FOR DISTRESS

Cancer Support Community Break Down Barriers To Care With Distress Screening—
    www.cancersupportcommunity.org/CancerSupportSource

Cancer Support Helpline—A free resource for people with cancer and their loved ones.
    Call with any question. 888-793-9355 or www.cancersupportcommunity.org/cancer
    -support-helpline

---

1. "Stress Weakens the Immune System," American Psychological Association, February 23, 2006, www.apa.org/research/action/immune.

CHAPTER 11

Ask About Fertility

Some cancers and their treatments may cause infertility in men and women. Infertility is the inability to conceive children. If you are trying to have a baby now or plan to at some point, this can be hard news to hear. It may come as a surprise. The impact of treatment on fertility depends on many factors, such as age, the type of treatment, and how long the treatment lasts. For example, some drugs can cause women to experience early menopause. Other treatments may affect a man's ability to produce healthy sperm.

Yet some people do go on to conceive children after being treated for cancer. There may be steps you can take now to increase the likelihood that you will be able to have biological children in the future. Fertility after cancer is still being studied. This area of research and treatment is referred to as oncofertility. It applies to both men and women.

It is very important to talk to your doctor as soon as possible, before treatment starts, if you plan to have children. Some, but not all, doctors will raise this topic with you as you discuss diagnosis and treatment. If your doctor does not mention it, be sure that you do. You may be able to preserve—or save—eggs, embryos, or sperm for future use.

This is called fertility preservation. There are several ways that this can be done. In some situations, it is possible to delay treatment for these procedures.

Fertility preservation is not an option for everyone. But when it is, common approaches include:[1]

Egg freezing: The process of freezing one or more unfertilized eggs to save them for future use. These are eggs that have not been combined with sperm. When it is time to use them, the eggs are thawed and fertilized in a lab to make embryos that can be placed in a woman's uterus. This is also called egg banking, egg cryopreservation, or oocyte cryopreservation.

Embryo freezing: The process of freezing one or more embryos to save them for future use. Embryo freezing involves in vitro fertilization. In this procedure, eggs are removed from a woman's ovary and combined with sperm in the lab to form embryos. The embryos are frozen and can later be thawed and placed in a woman's uterus. This is also called embryo banking or embryo cryopreservation.

Sperm freezing:[2] This is a simple process in which sperm are banked for future use. A man provides samples of his semen. A lab tests the sample for sperm count and health. Frozen sperm can be stored for many years.

Gonadal shielding: A procedure used during radiation therapy. A protective shield is placed on the outside of the body to cover the area of the gonads (the testicles or ovaries) and other parts of the reproductive system. For men, this would also include the prostate and penis. For women, it would also include the fallopian tubes, uterus, cervix, and vagina. This is sometimes called a radiation shield.

Your cancer team may refer you to a fertility doctor to explore your options. Doctors who specialize in this field are called reproductive endocrinologists. They are experts in hormone function, fertility, and fertility preservation. They can help you understand your options, the risks and benefits, and the rates of success.

---

1. Definitions adapted from the NCI Dictionary of Cancer Terms, National Cancer Institute, accessed October 20, 2020, www.cancer.gov/publications/dictionaries/cancer-terms.

2. "Male Fertility and Cancer," American Cancer Society, accessed October 20, 2020, www.cancer.org/treatment/treatments-and-side-effects/physical-side-effects/fertility-and-sexual-side-effects/fertility-and-men-with-cancer.html.

These procedures can be costly. Find out what your insurance will cover. Also, ask hospital staff members if they know of organizations in the hospital or community that can help with costs. Refer to the resources listed at the end of this chapter for more information.

You may feel like you already have too much on your mind to think about fertility. This is understandable. Fertility is just one of many things to consider as you develop your cancer treatment plan. In the "old days," doctors rarely raised these issues with patients and families, in part because the doctors themselves knew little about cancer and fertility. Often, a patient did not learn that they were infertile until months or years later, when they tried to start a family. Fortunately, we have come a long way since then. Today's guidelines recommend that doctors discuss fertility with any patient of child-bearing age. Doctors are encouraged to connect patients to specialists who can help think about and plan for a family after treatment ends.

If fertility is a priority for you, use the resources below to learn more. As you do, remember to ask for support. Fertility and cancer can raise a lot of questions and feelings. Look for people and groups that can help you talk through options, accept answers, and maintain perspective.

RESOURCES TO LEARN MORE ABOUT CANCER AND FERTILITY

Alliance for Fertility Preservation—Resource that covers all topics related to fertility preservation including approaches, risks, and cost. www.allianceforfertilitypreservation.org

American Cancer Society's "Fertility and Sexual Side Effects in People with Cancer"—Resource for learning more about fertility and cancer. www.cancer.org/treatment/treatments-and-side-effects/physical-side-effects/fertility-and-sexual-side-effects.html

Cancer Support Community's "Online Cancer Support"—Find support for thinking about fertility and other issues related to cancer. www.cancersupportcommunity.org/article/intimacy-sex-and-fertility-issues

Livestrong's "Becoming a Parent After Cancer"—Helps people with issues related to becoming a parent. www.livestrong.org/we-can-help/livestrong-fertility

Triage Cancer's "Quick Guide to Fertility Preservation"—A brief overview of fertility options including insurance coverage and cost. triagecancer.org/quickguide-fertility

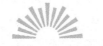

CHAPTER 12

Young Adults and Cancer

Being diagnosed with cancer at any age is very challenging. If you are young, you may feel even more shocked and overwhelmed by the sudden change in your life. This is normal. People in their late teens and into their twenties and thirties who have cancer face a unique set of challenges. Their physical and emotional needs are still not fully understood or addressed by the cancer care community.

For young adults, cancer can feel like an insurmountable hurdle. Young adults are generally defined as people ages eighteen to thirty-nine. At this stage of life, you may be focused on choosing or building a career, finding or nurturing romantic partnerships, deciding where and how to live, or starting a family. A cancer diagnosis can put plans on hold or take you in an entirely different direction.

At the Cancer Support Community, we support young adults by focusing on the issues unique to both their stage of life and their near- and long-term goals and aspirations. These include delayed diagnosis, dating, fertility, connecting with others going through the same experience, late- and long-term effects of treatment, and more. Let's look at some of these in more detail.

DELAYED DIAGNOSIS AND TREATMENT DECISIONS

Cancer is generally a disease of an aging population. It is rare for a young adult to be diagnosed with cancer. As a result, doctors often do not look for cancer right away when assessing a younger person's symptoms. If you were diagnosed with cancer at a young age or are close to someone who was, you may recall endless tests and appointments. Your doctor may have exhausted a long list of other possible diseases and ailments before they even considered cancer. They may have tried to treat your symptoms before ordering the tests that would have revealed cancer. If this sounds familiar, you are not alone.

If you find yourself in this situation now, this advice might be helpful:

- Listen to your body, be persistent, and be your own best advocate. You know when something is not right. Trust your instincts and keep looking until you find a doctor who will listen.

- Consider where you will be treated for cancer. Based on your age, you automatically fall into a unique category, and your case is considered rare. We strongly encourage you to do the research to find out who has experience treating both the type of cancer you have and people your age with this type of cancer. More and more, we see the emergence of specialists who have experience with young adults, especially at the larger academic centers. Even if you are over eighteen, it may still make sense to be treated at a children's hospital. Cancer in a young adult can look more like cancer in a child or may be a type of cancer more commonly found in children. In either of these situations, a children's hospital may be preferable. Refer to chapter three to learn more about building your health care team.

- Get a second opinion. Refer to chapter seven for more on why and how to do this.

- Explore clinical trials as an option for your care. A significant number of pediatric cancer patients are treated in clinical trials, as are some young adults. Be sure to learn about trials and ask your doctor if a clinical trial might be right for you. We cover clinical trials in greater detail in chapter eight.

MEDICAL ADHERENCE

Young people lead busy lives. And unlike older adults, whose lives sometimes revolve around health care, young adults are less accustomed to taking pills or having frequent medical appointments. As a result, they are not always adherent with their medications, appointments, and follow-up care. This is understandable but needs to be addressed.

When you are battling cancer, every dose and appointment counts. In order to have the best outcomes, it is critical that you adhere to your treatment schedule, medications, and all follow-up and surveillance appointments. Today, there are many apps and other technology solutions that can help. It can also help to connect with other young adult cancer survivors to get tips and advice on how to organize life with cancer.

CAREER DISRUPTION

Often, young adults are on a well-planned career trajectory. They may have set a goal to become a manager where they work or a partner at their firm in a set number of years or by a certain age. Or perhaps they have plans to start or complete a degree. Cancer can interrupt these plans. You may feel as if all your hard work and careful planning has been derailed.

It may be helpful to talk to your supervisor about your aspirations. Let them know that, while you may be away or have an altered schedule for a period of time, you remain committed. You still have ambitions for advancement and learning. It is also not unusual for cancer to lead to a reboot. After having cancer, you may decide to change direction and pursue a different career or set of goals.

While cancer may disrupt your plans, try to find the silver lining. Use this time for reflection. Look for meaning in the cancer experience. It may reframe how you view your life and your priorities, and perhaps have a profound impact on what you do next.

DATING AND INTIMACY

Young adults often find dating and intimacy a challenge during and after cancer. People with cancer have varying levels of openness or privacy about their health. Questions that might emerge include:

- When is the right time to tell someone you've met or are dating that you have cancer?

- How do you talk about the changes to your body? Or the limitations cancer may bring?

- How do changes to your body—whether from surgery or treatment—affect how you feel about your body and prompt you to think about how others may react?

- How does cancer affect your feelings about intimacy and sex?

- Could this information scare a potential partner away? Will people treat you differently now?

- How will the possible impact on future fertility affect your relationships?

Facing these questions can be scary—and make you feel uncertain. There are no right or clear answers or timelines. We can't predict how others will react to the news. Each person is different and operates on their own timetable. When and how you choose to share this information is up to you. It may help to talk to a therapist to work through your anxieties, or even to role-play possible conversations that you may have with a date or significant other. You may find it useful to connect with others your age who have had cancer. There are many ways to do this online or on social media. Know that you are not alone in facing these challenges. You can find people willing to have frank conversations and help you navigate these sensitive topics.

FERTILITY

Fertility can be a sensitive issue, even before cancer enters the picture. It is one of the top concerns of many young adults with cancer. There is some good news. Researchers have made great strides in fertility and cancer research. There are now options for fertility preservation and cancer treatment approaches that may limit the impact of cancer and its treatment on fertility. We discuss this topic in greater depth in chapter eleven.

CONNECTING WITH OTHERS

Young adults with cancer tell us that they really want to connect with people their age who have or have had cancer. If you are in your twenties or thirties, you may feel awkward or find that it is not helpful to be in a support group with folks in their sixties and seventies. They are at a completely different stage of life and may not relate to your concerns, nor you to theirs. The same may be true for cancer education programs. Fortunately, there are options. The increased recognition of the needs of young adults with cancer, coupled with the explosion of social media and digital connection, has filled a void. There are now a number of groups and advocacy and support organizations dedicated to the needs of young adults. Find others, connect, and seek out a safe place to share your fears, your concerns, and your hopes.

HEALTH INSURANCE AND THE GIG ECONOMY

Some young adults are part of the gig economy or work in places that do not offer health insurance. The gig economy is the growing part of the labor market characterized by freelance and contract work. People may work two or three different part-time or contract jobs. Some are self-employed and do not have health care coverage. If you are young, are diagnosed with cancer, and do not have health insurance, it is important to address this right away. In chapter nine, we discuss insurance and some steps you can take to seek coverage.

LATE-TERM EFFECTS

Because it is rare for young adults to be diagnosed with cancer, we do not know everything about the potential long-term impact of cancer treatment. As the field of cancer survivorship continues to emerge, we are learning more about the needs of patients after treatment and beyond. But there is still much to understand. Your doctor or nurse may invite you to join a study to follow you over years to monitor any symptoms and long-term effects. Consider doing this, both for your own health and as a way to help future generations.

Before you begin treatment, ask what is known about the long-term effects of different medications and procedures. Find out if there are strategies to minimize those effects. Be sure to monitor any symptoms or side effects that you experience, even if they are minor. Communicate with your doctors about these symptoms. A diligent long-term care plan will help with long-term survivorship, recovery, and outcomes.

After the cancer has been treated and the oncologist has discharged you from the cancer clinic, it is critical to continue to see a primary care doctor. They can help monitor your health for long-term effects of the cancer treatment.

If you are a young adult diagnosed with cancer, ask lots of questions, find the right treatment center and team, and connect with other young adults who are having similar experiences. At the end of this chapter, we list some excellent resources to help you navigate cancer and find a community of support tailored to you.

"I was twenty-nine years old when I was diagnosed in 2000. I thought my life was over. I thought, this is it, nobody is going to want me, I'm not going to have a long life to live, I'm not going to see my nieces and nephews grow up. I wasn't married at the time and I will say, looking back on all of this, I found a wonderful husband. I have had great family support and friends. Your view of life changes. You don't sweat the small stuff as much. When I start feeling bad, I just remember there are other people who have had it worse and I'm thankful to be here."

—Christy, head and neck cancer survivor

Out Living It

BRAD LUDDEN, FOUNDER OF FIRST DESCENTS

Inspired by his aunt's battle with breast cancer, Brad Ludden, a professional kayaker, created First Descents to offer life-changing outdoor adventures for young adults impacted by cancer and other serious health conditions.

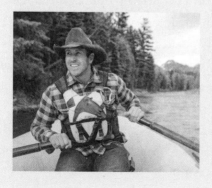

In the face of a rapid, we are all equal. The river doesn't care about our past, our successes or failures, our job, our zip code, or the color of our skin. She treats us all the same, cancer or not. This leveled playing field—albeit peppered with rapids and beauty and boulders and horizon lines—creates heightened feelings of fear, success, failure, and friendship. At the bottom of the rapid, in our kayaks, we know that we earned it; that the river didn't give any of us a break. She merely opened the door and we paddled through it—both as individuals and as a team.

For as long as I can remember, I've sought outdoor adventures. For years I did it because it was all I knew. I was raised in the outdoors—hiking, camping, hunting, kayaking, skiing, and just generally chasing a good adventure. This went from a passion to a profession in my teens when I became a sponsored white-water kayak athlete. I spent the next two decades traveling around the world in search of remote rivers that had never been kayaked before. During those years I found myself forming friendships that felt more like family. Friendships that, to this day, are at the very foundation of my life. The community that was built on the river has carried me through hard times, provided endless laughter and lessons, and is always there at a moment's notice. In short, and without knowing it, the river gave me one of my life's greatest gifts, my closest friends.

Somewhere along the way, I decided that the healing power of adventure, and the support systems that rise from it, from which I had so greatly bene-fited, needed to be shared with others. That's when I decided to start First Descents (FD)—an organization that provides outdoor adventures to young adults impacted by cancer and other serious health conditions.

Immediately after founding First Descents we began to hear a consistent theme from our participants: "I just felt so alone after my diagnosis. I had a lot of people who cared about me and were there throughout, but try as they might, they just couldn't relate." It's those feelings of isolation that often lead young adults to FD. They're in search of their people—their community—in search of people who've lived through what they did and can relate on a level others cannot. They want to be able to share stories, ask questions, laugh, connect, and be understood. It's that shared experience of cancer that brings them to FD and begins to build a deep connection, and it's their shared FD adventure that forges it in stone.

That community has grown to thousands of young adults over the past twenty years, from all corners of the world and all walks of life. It's full of young adults who are now adventuring and connecting together all over the country, every day. We have a saying at FD: we're *Out Living It*. I couldn't think of a better way to describe this community and the ethos upon which it stands—defiantly, and together, adventuring in the face of adversity. We are Out Living It, and we want you to join us.

Let the adventure begin . . .

RESOURCES FOR YOUNG ADULTS WITH CANCER

Cancer Support Community Blog—Essays by young adults with cancer that address a range of topics. www.cancersupportcommunity.org/blog

First Descents—Provides life-changing outdoor adventures for young adults (ages eighteen to thirty-nine) impacted by cancer and other serious health conditions. www .firstdescents.org

Living Beyond Breast Cancer's Young Women's Initiative—Support and resources for women diagnosed before age forty-five. 888-753-5222 or www.lbbc.org/young -womens-initiative

Stupid Cancer—A community of young adults affected by cancer. stupidcancer.org

Ulman Cancer Fund—Support and resources for young adults affected by cancer and their loved ones. ulmanfoundation.org

Young Survival Coalition—Resources, connections, and outreach for young women with breast cancer. 877-972-1011 or www.youngsurvival.org

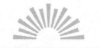

CHAPTER 13

Set Up Advance Directives

Let's face it—nobody wants to talk about living wills, health care proxies, and do-not-resuscitate orders, even when they are well. It can be harder when facing a serious illness. You or your loved ones may feel stressed or upset. It may feel like giving up. But these tools will allow you to take some control over your situation. They will give your loved ones guidance and peace of mind, should they need to make decisions on your behalf. Putting these tools in place will be a gift to your family in a time of relative uncertainty. We've all heard stories of siblings fighting because everyone thinks they know what a parent would want, or of a spouse unable to act in the face of such daunting decisions. By being proactive now, you can help reduce confusion and conflict among your loved ones. You can be clear about your wishes.

What are advance directives? According to *Merriam-Webster's Dictionary*, an advance directive is "a legal document, such as a living will, signed by a competent person to provide guidance for medical and health care decisions, such as the termination of life support or organ donation, in the event the person becomes incompetent to make such decisions." These documents ensure that someone you trust can make decisions on your behalf if you are unable to do so. It is important to think about who this might be and try to have these documents in order as you begin treatment. This area is also called advance care planning.

"It was a great relief to make our wishes known. It took a lot of pressure off."
—Pete, acute myelemia leukemia survivor

—

Let's dig a little deeper into these documents and how you can prepare them:[1]

Living will: This document states the kind of medical treatment you would want if you were no longer able to make your wishes known. It lists different kinds of care, such as breathing tubes, feeding tubes, and CPR. You specify which ones you would want or not want. In the past, this was sometimes called an advance directive. Now that term is used more broadly to refer to the group of documents listed here. A living will is one kind of advance directive. The laws related to living wills vary by state. Not every state honors them.

Durable power of attorney for health care: This document gives permission to a trusted person you choose to make decisions on your behalf. This person can speak for you when you are not able. This is also called a health care proxy or medical power of attorney.

Do-not-resuscitate order: This is an order that a doctor writes in your chart. It reminds your doctors and other members of your health care team of how you would like them to act if your heart or lungs stop working. Do you want to be put on machines if your body cannot stay alive on its own? Discuss this with your family so that they know your wishes.

Many people ask, "How do I start putting these documents in place? Do I need a lawyer? Is it going to be expensive?" The bottom line is no—you generally do not need a lawyer. Many of these documents are available online and may simply require you to complete and sign them. But it is important to note that advance directive laws vary by

---

1. NCI Dictionary of Cancer Terms, National Cancer Institute, www.cancer.gov/publications /dictionaries/cancer-terms.

state. Some states require the signature of a witness or notary public. Others may have different requirements. Be sure to use the correct documents for your state and follow its guidelines to make sure that your wishes will be honored.

ADVANCE CARE PLANNING CHECKLIST[2]

❏ Have I discussed advance care planning with my family and health care team?

❏ Have I documented my wishes in a legally suitable format?

❏ Have I legally chosen someone to make medical decisions for me in case I cannot do so myself?

❏ When was the last time I reviewed all my documents that detail my wishes?

❏ Do my loved ones and health care team have a copy and know where my documents are?

2. Cancer Support Community, *Frankly Speaking About Cancer: Metastatic Breast Cancer*, February 2019, www.cancersupportcommunity.org/sites/default /files/fields/resource/file/2018-03/mbc_book_2018.pdf.

RESOURCES FOR ADVANCE CARE PLANNING

Cancer Support Community's "Legal Concerns and Cancer"—A list of legal documents to have in place. www.cancersupportcommunity.org/legal-concerns-cancer

The Conversation Project—Resources to help you start talking about your end-of-life wishes. www.theconversationproject.org

NHPCO (National Hospice and Palliative Care Organization)—Offers downloadable advance directives forms for each state. www.nhpco.org/patients-and-caregivers /advance-care-planning/advance-directives/downloading-your-states-advance -directive/

Triage Cancer—Learn more about the documents in this chapter. triagecancer.org

CHAPTER 14

Care for the Caregiver

If you are the caregiver or loved one of someone with cancer, this book is for you, too. You may benefit from the information and encouragement found throughout its pages, but this chapter is especially for you. It is geared toward your needs as a caregiver. These tips will help you **take care of yourself** while taking care of your loved one.

When your loved one is diagnosed with cancer, you are thrust into a role for which you probably have had no training or background. Just managing the emotions associated with your loved one's cancer can be overwhelming and scary. On top of that, you may be helping with research, gathering medical information, finding doctors, imagining the impact on your family's finances, taking care of children and other family members, and more. You also may be frightened about losing your loved one.

So, what does it mean to be a caregiver? What do caregivers do? The Cancer Support Community's Cancer Experience Registry is a research study that examines the experiences of cancer patients and caregivers.[1] We asked caregivers to tell us the tasks they have taken on since becoming caregivers. More than six hundred cancer caregivers responded. Here is what they shared:

- 96 percent provided emotional support.
- 91 percent went with their loved one to medical appointments.
- 79 percent helped with decision-making.
- 78 percent coordinated medical care.
- 78 percent provided transportation.
- 69 percent helped manage finances.

And this is only a partial list. Caregivers do these things out of love or obligation, or because there is no one else. You may feel like it's all on you. If you feel this way, you are not alone, and you don't have to take on all these tasks alone. Now is the time to get help and seek support.

———————

"I feel that the word caregiver *falls short of describing the breadth of my role as a true partner in this fight. Cancer is a huge, life-changing event that deeply affects not only the patient, but those closest to them. Andy and I are in this together every step of the way—we love and support each other; we give each other strength and hope."*
—Jeanne, caregiver of a loved one with acute myeloid leukemia

———————

GET HELP

If you can, engage other family members, friends, and your health care team in the care of your loved one. Ask them for help and advice. There are many ways to do this. Some people give friends and family specific tasks and assignments. For example, you may ask

———————

1. "Cancer Experience Registry," Cancer Support Community, accessed November 17, 2020, www.cancerexperienceregistry.org.

one person to research doctors, treatments, and clinical trials. You may ask someone else to get answers to financial and insurance questions. Others may provide rides to treatment, help with food preparation and meal delivery, or assist with the kids. There are many apps and websites you can use to ask for and organize help. You may find that people around you want to help and are happy to be given jobs to support you.

You will likely have times when you feel overwhelmed as a caregiver. You may feel like the clock never stops, and you may feel guilty for stepping away and doing something for yourself. But it's important to realize that caring for yourself—even in small doses—helps you be the best caregiver you can be for your loved one.

"We feel guilty when we do something for ourselves, even going to work. We try to be by their sides all the time but that can take a toll."
—Devon, caregiver of a loved one with tonsil cancer

There are many ways you can take care of yourself. Plan breaks. Connect with friends. Go outside and get some fresh air. Taking time for you will help keep everyone on track, help reduce stress, and remind you that the little things matter.

What happens when you do not live near your loved ones? You face the challenge of caregiving from a distance. This can be frustrating and can lead to feelings of guilt and separation from others. There are many ways to support your loved one, even if you are not nearby.[2] You can:

- help build a support team of friends and family who are geographically close to your loved one.
- use technology to connect with your loved one and participate in meetings with doctors and care providers.
- arrange for home care providers or companions to check in on your loved one and help with tasks like bathing, dressing, and meals.
- make sure someone is available and nearby to help in an emergency or crisis—even a kind neighbor. You will continue to be surprised by how many people want to help.

---

2. Cancer Support Community, *Frankly Speaking About Cancer: Support from a Distance*, 2011, www.cancersupportcommunity.org/support-distance.

TAKE A BREAK[3]

Be sure to put some planned breaks on your calendar.
If you feel yourself getting anxious, tired, or distracted, try taking a
mini-break.
Here are some ideas:

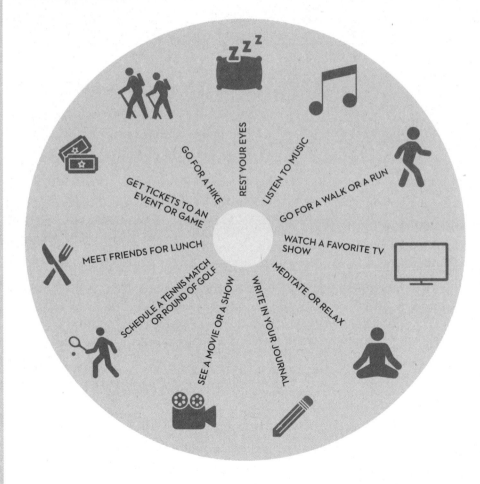

---

3. Cancer Support Community, *Frankly Speaking About Cancer: Caregivers*, May
2020, www.cancersupportcommunity.org/caregivers.

"Don't lose sight of yourself. It's easy to get wrapped up in the process of appointments and waiting. Don't get caught up. Take even five minutes to find out what you need for yourself. It's not easy, but you have to take care of yourself, too."
—Sarah, caregiver of a loved one with brain cancer

SEEK SUPPORT

Being a caregiver puts you close to a stressful and scary situation, one that may affect your life personally. You may worry about your loved one's health, the work you are missing to care for them, and the impact their illness has on you or your family's future and finances.

There are people and services that can help you as you help your loved one. Here, we focus on the importance of seeking emotional support. Feeling better mentally may make it easier to handle the business of life. At the end of this chapter, we include resources to help with work, money, and other life challenges.

CAREGIVERS NEED TO KNOW

The *Family and Medical Leave Act (FMLA)* allows an ill person or family member caring for them to take up to twelve weeks off from work (without pay but with no loss of benefits). Time off can be taken a little at a time or all at once.[4]

Respite care is organized short-term care that makes it possible for a caregiver to take a break from the daily routine and stress of caregiving. Take time to learn about the respite care services near you.[5]

---

4. Cancer Support Community, *Frankly Speaking: Caregivers*.
5. Cancer Support Community, *Frankly Speaking: Caregivers*.

Many caregivers find it helpful to join a support group, either in person or online, where they can connect with other caregivers. Caregiver support groups can help you:

- feel less alone and isolated.
- solve problems and ask others for tips and advice.
- open up in a private setting about feelings, emotions, fears, and anxieties.
- learn about new resources in your local hospital or community.
- manage some of the stresses of being a caregiver.
- improve coping skills.

If you feel like support groups are not for you, look for other forms of support. Some caregivers find it helpful to talk one-on-one with a social worker, counselor, psychologist, or clergyperson. Others appreciate the support of friends or family members, perhaps those who are less involved with your loved one. If you are not sure where to find help, talk with your loved one's health care team or use the resources listed at the end of this chapter. The Cancer Support Helpline (888-793-9355) is here for you as well.

Whether you are nearby or farther away, it is important to discuss with your loved one what role they want you to play, and for you to respect their wishes. This may be difficult, especially if you don't agree with their choices. As a person with cancer, they need to regain some control over their own life. One of the ways this happens is that they make decisions about their own care and treatment.

"As a caregiver, you can help find information, but remember that it is the person going through the cancer who makes the ultimate decision. It's their cancer plan. It is their treatment. You need to support whatever decision they make."
—Terese, caregiver of a loved one with bladder cancer

Caregiving is not all work and stress. You may find some satisfaction in the role. Caregiving can help you feel closer to your loved one and other family members. It may bring a deeper purpose to your life. You may get to know your loved one better by spending more time with them and hearing personal stories and memories. You may use this time to work together, planning for the future—perhaps a graduation or wedding weeks or months away—or a special activity next week or even tomorrow. Try to find gratitude in caring for another human being, and look for ways to bring your unique talents, skills, and personality to the role.

———————

"As a caregiver, you have to give 100 percent. You have to be organized, take notes, and understand what is happening."
—Benny, caregiver of a loved one with acute lymphoblastic leukemia

———————

RESOURCES FOR CAREGIVERS

ARCH National Respite Network and Resource Center—Provides respite to caregivers. www.archrespite.org

Cancer Support Community's *Caregivers* page—www.cancersupportcommunity.org /caregivers

Cancer Support Community's *Frankly Speaking About Cancer: Support from a Distance*— www.cancersupportcommunity.org/support-distance

Caregiver Action Network—Education, peer support, and resources for caregivers. www .caregiveraction.org

Family Caregiver Alliance—Support and resources for caregivers. www.caregiver.org

National Alliance for Caregiving—Resources and advocacy related to caregiving. www .caregiving.org

Rosalynn Carter Institute for Caregiving—Building support for caregivers worldwide. www.rosalynncarter.org

SECTION TWO

ACTIVE TREATMENT

CHAPTER 15

Time to Gear Up for Treatment

You have completed all diagnostic tests, received your diagnosis, and have a sense of your treatment plan and schedule. In all likelihood, you have been given a lot of information. If you've got it all organized in one place, give yourself a high five. That's impressive! If you're like most of us, you have scribbled on scraps of paper here and there or have some notes on your computer or your phone.

This chapter is designed to help you organize your diagnosis and treatment information in one place. You can even take this book with you to medical appointments. There is a place in the back to jot down notes and questions. Start filling in the details below to the best of your ability. It's okay if you don't know everything. Record what you know and fill in the blanks as you go along.

Fill in the information about your cancer diagnosis and treatment below:

Type and Subtype of Cancer: _____

Stage of Cancer: _____

Positive Biomarkers: _____

Name of Treatment Center: _____

Address of Treatment Center: _____

    Fill in your medications and doses:

Brand Name of Medicine: _____ _____

Generic Name of Medicine: _____

Dose of Medicine: _____

Way Medication Is Administered (oral, IV, injection, etc.): _____

Number of Times Treatment Will Be Given: _____

Time or Interval Between Treatments: _____

Brand Name of Medicine: _____

Generic Name of Medicine: _____

Dose of Medicine: _____

Way Medication Is Administered (oral, IV, injection, etc.): _____

Number of Times Treatment Will Be Given: _____

Time or Interval Between Treatments: _____

Brand Name of Medicine: _____

Generic Name of Medicine: _____

Dose of Medicine: _____

Way Medication Is Administered (oral, IV, injection, etc.): _____

Number of Times Treatment Will Be Given: _____

Time or Interval Between Treatments: _____

Here you can list your doctors and nurses and their contact information. Ask them if it is possible to email with questions:

Name of Doctor: _____

Type of Doctor (medical oncologist, surgeon, radiation oncologist, etc.): _____

_____

Name of Nurse: _____

Office Phone Number: _____

Office Address: _____

Email Addresses: _____

Name of Doctor: _____

Type of Doctor (medical oncologist, surgeon, radiation oncologist, etc.): _____

_____

Name of Nurse: _____

Office Phone Number: _____

Office Address: _____

Email Addresses: _____

Name of Doctor: _____

Type of Doctor (medical oncologist, surgeon, radiation oncologist, etc.): _____

_____

Name of Nurse: _____

Office Phone Number: _____

Office Address: _____

Email Addresses: _____

Names of other care providers (social worker, registered dietician, physical therapist, genetic counselor, etc.):

Name: _____

Area of Specialty: _____

Phone Number: _____

Office Address: ____   _____

Email: _____

Name: _____

Area of Specialty: _____

Phone Number: _____

Office Address: _____

Email: _____

Name: _____

Area of Specialty: _____

Phone Number: _____

Office Address: _____

Email: _____

Name: _____

Area of Specialty: _____

Phone Number: _____

Office Address: _____

Email: _____

Add other important information to have handy and in one place:

Name of Insurance Provider: _____

Phone Number of Insurance Provider: _____

Group Number: _____

Member Number: _____

Name of Secondary Insurance Provider: _____

Phone Number of Secondary Insurance Provider: _____

Group Number: _____

Member Number: _____

Name of Support Group: _____

Location of Support Group: _____

Contact Phone Number for Support Group: _____

Date, Time, and Frequency of Support Group: _____

Name of Private Counselor or Therapist: _____

Phone Number: _____

Email: _____

NOTES: _____

_____

_____

_____

_____

_____

_____

_____

_____

_____

_____

_____

"It's a good thing I asked about immunotherapy. Asking that question saved my life."
—Karl, bladder cancer survivor

RESOURCES TO KEEP TRACK OF MEDICAL INFORMATION

American Cancer Society's "My Medicines Form"—A printable form you can use to keep track of medication you are taking. www.cancer.org/content/dam/cancer-org/cancer -control/en/worksheets/medicine-list.pdf

Cancer Support Community's "Cancer Diagnosis? What You Need to Know"— Everything you need to know when facing a cancer diagnosis. www.cancersupport community.org/cancer-diagnosis-what-you-need-know

Cancer Support Community's "Cancer Treatment Side Effects"—A go-to resource for managing specific side effects. www.cancersupportcommunity.org/cancer-treatment -side-effects

Recommended mobile apps to help you keep track of medications, side effects, appointments, and more:

CancerAid app—www.canceraid.com
Cancer.Net Mobile app—www.cancer.net/navigating-cancer-care/managing-your-care /cancernet-mobile

CHAPTER 16

Learn How to Manage Side Effects

Everyone knows that cancer treatment can cause side effects. The potential side effects vary by type of treatment, and the experience varies from person to person. Some of the better known side effects include hair loss, nausea, vomiting, fatigue, and infection. Newer drugs can cause skin rash or flu-like symptoms.

The good news is that doctors have come a long way in managing side effects and taking steps to prevent or lessen their severity. It is important to talk with your medical team about side effects. Ask about the possible side effects of every treatment you consider. Find out if there are ways to plan for and preempt them and what you can do if these side effects arise. For example:

- At what point do you call or email the doctor or nurse?
- Are there over-the-counter medications that can help?
- When do you go to the emergency room?

Since some side effects can be severe and even life-threatening, please do not suffer in silence. There are ways to manage side effects and perhaps even options you haven't considered. Your doctor may be able to give you a temporary "holiday" from treatment or reduce the dose of the drugs you are taking so you can better tolerate the treatment. Good preparation and a contingency plan can help ease your mind and let your caregivers know what to look for and how to help.

COPING WITH SIDE EFFECTS[1]

Lists of possible side effects are long and can be scary to think about. For some, coping with side effects is one of the hardest parts of having cancer. Keep in mind:

- You probably will not have all the side effects mentioned. Each person reacts differently to treatment. Some people get through treatment with very mild side effects.
- Your health care team can help you manage side effects. They can offer tips to prevent side effects and recommend or prescribe medicines that can help.
- Your health care team knows only what you tell them. Tell your health care team about any changes you notice. They can help you only if they know what is going on.
- There are new ways to treat and prevent side effects. If you had a bad experience with a certain side effect before, you may worry about managing it. Doctors continue to study side effect management. There may be new strategies or better medicines.
- You are not alone. Talking with other people who have been on the same drugs can be very helpful. You may find them in a support group or through your health care team.

---

1. Cancer Support Community, *Frankly Speaking About Cancer: Metastatic Breast Cancer*, February 2019, www.cancersupportcommunity.org/mbc.

"I had responded to chemo so well that I went into [bone marrow] transplant with a superhero complex. The transplant was no joke. When I got home, I started to feel the effects. The doctor warned me, but I didn't realize how much it would affect me."
—Jen, acute myeloid leukemia survivor

In this chapter, we outline some of the most common side effects of cancer treatment, what to look for, and how they are managed.[2]

Anemia, infection, and bleeding: Cancer treatments can affect your red blood cell, white blood cell, and platelet counts. Low levels of red blood cells can cause anemia and fatigue. Low levels of white blood cells can increase your risk of infection. Treatment can also affect your body's level of platelets—the cells that allow your body to form blood clots when needed. Low levels of platelets can lead to easy bruising or bleeding. Your health care team will monitor your blood counts and tell you what signs to look for. Your team can help you manage symptoms of anemia and give you tips to prevent infection and bleeding. For example, it may be helpful to eat foods rich in iron and get rest. Wash your hands and avoid being around people who are sick to prevent infection. Try to avoid injury, and take care when brushing your teeth to prevent bleeding. In some situations, blood transfusions are used to increase blood cells counts.

Cognitive changes ("chemo brain"): Chemotherapy can cause changes to your thinking. You may feel forgetful, become confused, or have trouble recalling words. It can help to make lists and write things down. Let the people around you know what you are experiencing. They can be more helpful and patient.

---

2. Cancer Support Community, *Frankly Speaking About Cancer: Coping with Side Effects*, December 2019, www.cancersupportcommunity.org/sites/default/files/fields/resource/file/2020 -01/coping_with_side_effects_book.pdf.

"The radiation has affected my memory. I have to keep lists of everything or I forget. And I keep a journal and write down everything that I did during the day. Before I go to bed, I can refer back to it if I need to remember something. If I don't write it down, it's just like it didn't happen, and so partly I write it down just to have a record of my life because I don't remember past about twenty-four hours. I make lists all the time, all day long—I have Post-it notes everywhere just to remind myself of what I need to do. That's another coping strategy."
—Christy, head and neck cancer survivor

Constipation: Chemotherapy and drugs used to treat pain can interfere with regular bowel movements. You also may be prone to this if you are less active. If this is a possible side effect of treatment, start drinking more fluids and changing your diet in advance to prevent it. There are also medicines that can help.

Diarrhea: Certain drugs may cause very loose or watery stools. There are changes you can make to your diet to help prevent and manage diarrhea. For example, you can avoid caffeine and spicy foods, and eat smaller meals. If you have more than three incidents of diarrhea in a day, call your health care team.

Fatigue: Fatigue is one of the most common side effects of cancer treatment. It is a feeling of tiredness that you just can't shake. Keep track of when you feel the most tired and how long it lasts. Notice when you have energy and use that time. Take good care of your body—try to sleep, exercise, drink water, and eat healthy foods.

"Fatigue has been a big part of the disease since day one. I can't shake it, whether it's from the disease, medication, or aging. It's like you hit a brick wall."
—Diane, chronic myeloid leukemia survivor

Hair loss: Some chemo drugs can cause hair loss in some people. You may lose hair on any or all parts of your body. Hair may start to fall out ten to twenty-one days after you start treatment. There are many ways to prepare for and deal with hair loss, including the use of a cooling cap to help prevent it. Be sure to find out what your insurance will cover.

Hot flashes: Hormone treatments can cause hot flashes, as well as vaginal dryness and other symptoms of menopause. It can help to exercise, wear lighter clothing and layers, and avoid hot showers, spicy foods, alcohol, and smoking. Acupuncture is sometimes used to relieve symptoms.

Infertility: Refer to chapter eleven for more on fertility and cancer.

Lymphedema: Treatment can damage the lymph nodes, causing swelling and pain in the extremities. It often occurs in the arms and hands. There are many steps you can take to manage it and reduce pain, including exercising, wearing a compression sleeve, and avoiding lifting heavy objects. You might want to ask your care team for a referral to a clinic that treats lymphedema.

Mouth and throat problems: Certain drugs and radiation can affect your mouth and interfere with eating. You may develop mouth sores, dry mouth, or changes to your sense of taste or smell. Depending on the problem, there are treatments and strategies to help, like avoiding hot foods or using plastic utensils. You may find relief in ice chips or chewing gum.

"The doctor gave me a rinse. I was constantly rinsing, which had a numbing effect. There were a couple of days when I couldn't eat at all or take my pills. I couldn't even swallow my own saliva. My doctor prescribed a narcotic for the pain. I tried not to take anything because you hear so much about people getting dependent. Then I realized that it was better to take some pain medicine and be able to eat a little and take my pills."
—Laura on coping with mouth sores, a side effect of treatment for multiple myeloma

---

Nausea and vomiting: Nausea is a common side effect of cancer treatment. There are many drugs you can take to prevent and treat nausea. People also find relaxation exercises such as meditation and deep breathing to be helpful.

Nerve problems (neuropathy): You may notice pain, tingling, swelling, or muscle weakness. It often begins in the hands or feet. Let your health care team know if you have new pain, if you are not able to feel the ground when you walk, or if you have trouble lifting small objects or buttoning a shirt.

Pain: Pain has many possible causes. If you have pain, keep track of where it is, what it feels like, when you notice it, and how long it lasts. Also note the severity of pain on a scale of one to ten with ten being the worst. Talk with your health care team and keep track of anything you take to treat pain. There are many ways to manage pain, and pain can get worse if it is not managed. Tell your team about any pain you have.

Sexual side effects: Refer to chapter twenty-three for more on how cancer and cancer treatment can affect sexuality, and tips to manage.

Skin and nail changes and rashes: Certain drugs and radiation can cause changes that affect the skin. Changes vary by treatment but can include redness, dryness, itching, burning, pain, or rashes. There may be ways to prevent this. Ask your doctor in advance. It is also helpful to report any changes you notice right away and ask about treatment. This is especially true if you are taking targeted therapy. If left untreated, skin and nail problems can become severe. Likewise, changes to the hands and feet caused by chemotherapy may be a sign of hand-foot syndrome and should be treated right away.

"I know that the side effects are manageable. They are pretty much annoying, but they are manageable. I do get mouth sores, and I have a magic mouthwash that was prescribed. I get pain in my right side that lasts maybe three days. The fatigue is pretty much the most of it. Brittle nails and thinning hair . . . I started taking biotin for my nails, so they have just started getting better. The hair, not so much. But the way that I cope with them is I know that they are only temporary, so it's easy to get through."
—Lynn, chronic lymphocytic leukemia survivor

Sleep changes: Your body needs rest to fight cancer. If you find that you are unable to fall asleep or you wake in the middle of the night, focus on improving your sleep habits. For example, avoid caffeine and stick to a regular bedtime routine. If worry keeps you awake, try relaxing with meditation or seek support from a therapist. If the problem becomes severe, your doctor may prescribe medicine to help.

Urinary and bladder problems: These can include inability to urinate, blood in the urine, painful urination, leaking, cloudy or red urine, and infection. They may be accompanied by back pain or fever. Be sure to report these symptoms early on to prevent or treat infection.

Weight changes: Cancer can affect your weight in different ways. Treatment can make it harder to eat or hold down food, leading to weight loss. Or you may find that discomfort or fatigue interferes with your activity level, causing weight gain. Changes in weight can affect how we feel about ourselves and our overall health. Talk with your doctor about your concerns and how to address them.

On the next page, there is a chart you can photocopy and use to track your side effects on a daily basis.

Type of Treatment	Most Common Side Effects
Chemotherapy	Anemia (low red blood cell count); cognitive changes; constipation; diarrhea; fatigue; hair loss; low white blood cell and platelet counts; mouth sores; nail and skin changes; nausea; numbness or tingling in the hands or feet; taste changes; vomiting; weight loss
Hormone therapy	Hot flashes; menopausal symptoms; muscle and bone pain; tiredness; vaginal dryness
Immunotherapy	Flu-like symptoms (fever, chills, dizziness, muscle aches, nausea, weakness, headache, etc.); diarrhea; fatigue; muscle or joint pain; skin reactions (like rash, redness, or itching); swelling and weight gain
Radiation therapy	Fatigue; skin changes; nausea; long-term side effects
Surgery	Pain; fatigue; appetite loss; swelling, bruising, or bleeding near the site
Targeted therapy	Blurry vision; diarrhea; fatigue; loss of appetite; low blood counts; mouth sores; nail infection; skin changes; skin rash

Side Effect	
Date/Time	Notes
Date/Time	
Date/Time	

Side Effect	
Date/Time	Notes
Date/Time	
Date/Time	

Side Effect	
Date/Time	Notes
Date/Time	
Date/Time	

Side Effect	
Date/Time	Notes
Date/Time	
Date/Time	

GENERAL TIPS TO HELP MANAGE SIDE EFFECTS[3]

- *Eat healthy foods.* Good nutrition maintains energy, strengthens the immune system, and can decrease side effects.
- *Drink liquids.* Adequate fluid intake prevents dehydration, helps decrease constipation, and decreases fatigue.
- *Try to do some physical activity every day.* Exercise combats fatigue, promotes restful sleep, and can elevate your mood. Ask your health care team which exercises may help you.
- *Tell your health care team about all medicines you are taking.* This includes drugs that have been prescribed and over-the-counter ones like aspirin, cold remedies, vitamins, or herbal supplements. Some medicines and combinations of medicines can cause side effects or make them worse. Some can even interfere with your treatment.
- *Wash your hands to decrease the risk of infection.* Ask family members and friends to do the same. Avoid having visitors who are sick or are exposed to young children who are sick.
- *Try to relax.* Yoga, meditation, and deep breathing can help reduce stress and increase energy.
- *Seek support.* Talking with others can help you understand and manage your feelings.
- *Tell your doctor and nurse about any changes you notice.* They may be side effects. Your health care team has resources and techniques to help you manage them.

---

3. Adapted from Cancer Support Community, *Frankly Speaking About Cancer: Coping with Side Effects*, December 2019, www.cancersupport community.org/cancer-treatment-side-effects.

ASK ABOUT PALLIATIVE CARE

Palliative care is an area of medicine that focuses on improving quality of life. It is provided by specially trained doctors and nurses. They work with your other doctors to help manage the symptoms of cancer or the side effects of treatment. It is sometimes confused with hospice care, but they are not the same. Today, palliative care is appropriate for someone with any stage of cancer. Ask if your hospital or cancer center has a palliative care specialist.

Living Longer and Better Thanks to Palliative Care

AMY BERMAN, RN, LHD, FAAN

Amy Berman, RN, has been living with stage IV breast cancer for a decade. She is a senior program officer for the John A. Hartford Foundation in New York City, working to improve care for older adults.

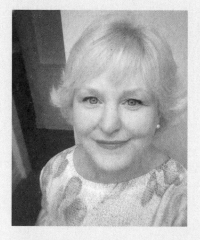

It's been nearly ten years since I was diagnosed with cancer. I still remember the day I saw a red spot on my right breast. The area was puckered like the peel of an orange. Because I am a nurse, I recognized it as a telltale sign of inflammatory breast cancer, the deadliest form of breast cancer. After a mammogram, biopsy, and scan, the oncologist confirmed that it was in fact inflammatory breast cancer and it was stage IV, spread to my lower spine. I was devastated. I felt fine, but I had advanced cancer.

I cared about what was to come. How long might I live? How would I feel? According to the National Cancer Institute, the prognosis, the likely course of the disease, was that 11 to 20 percent of people with my condition survived for five years. In other words, it was highly unlikely that I would live five years. Yet here I am, almost ten years later, still alive, working, and having fun-filled adventures.

How do I live well in the face of serious illness? I have a secret weapon called palliative care. Before I tell you what palliative care is, I want to share what palliative care has done for me. I'm an adventurer. I love traveling with friends and family. Since being diagnosed, I have climbed the Great Wall of China, ridden a jet ski in New York Harbor, gone camel riding in the Jordanian desert, swum in Coney Island's freezing waters on New Year's Day with the Polar Bear Club, and snowmobiled on a glacier in the Arctic Circle. I also continue to work every day and love what I do.

Palliative care has allowed me to keep living a great life in the face of advanced cancer. Palliative care is an extra layer of support that goes along with the usual care and treatment I receive. There is a team of specially trained doctors, nurses, and social workers and even a chaplain that provide palliative care. They focus on managing pain and symptoms, coordinating care, supporting the family, and addressing spiritual needs.

Here is an example of what the palliative care team did for me.

Around four or five years ago, I felt a pain in my back just under my right shoulder blade. It hurt when I moved my arm. It hurt a lot when I rode the subway and held onto an overhead handle. I thought that I might have a small fracture. The X-ray was clear. But the follow-up scan showed that cancer was in my ribs next to the spine. The pain was wearing on me. Since I was working and could tolerate the pain, I avoided taking medications to make me feel better. But this strategy wasn't working. I was miserable.

The standard treatment for pain from bone metastasis is ten to twenty doses of radiation. It doesn't cure the cancer. It gets rid of the pain. I went to see my palliative care clinician, who said a new study showed that one larger dose of radiation can be as effective as ten to twenty regular doses. That means the pain would go away quicker and I could have less redness, peeling skin, loss of appetite, and tiredness. It is called single-fraction radiation (one dose that's larger). I opted for single-fraction radiation and it turned off the pain like a light switch. My skin wasn't red. No peeling. I felt fine—no, I felt *great*! The next day I took the train to Washington, DC.

I can't share all the ways that palliative care has helped me these past nine and a half years, but if you met me, you would see I live a great life and, thankfully, a longer life. If you want to find the palliative care team in your area, go to www.getpalliativecare.org.

RESOURCES TO LEARN MORE ABOUT SIDE EFFECTS AND HOW TO COPE WITH THEM

Use these resources to look up specific side effects and how to manage them:

American Cancer Society's "Treatments and Side Effects"—www.cancer.org/treatment/treatments-and-side-effects.html

American Society of Clinical Oncologists—cancer.net

Cancer Support Community's "Cancer Treatment Side Effects"—Links to many helpful resources, including an essential planner and a detailed book on side effects and how to manage them. www.cancersupportcommunity.org/cancer-treatment-side-effects

- Cancer Support Community's *Frankly Speaking About Cancer: Coping with Side Effects*—Learn more about managing side effects with this in-depth book.
- Cancer Support Community's "Coping with Side Effects Planner"—A rich resource for keeping track of treatment and side effects in detail.

National Cancer Institute's "Side Effects of Cancer Treatment"—www.cancer.gov/about-cancer/treatment/side-effects

CHAPTER 17

Talking to Your Kids About Cancer

At the Cancer Support Community, we see more and more people with cancer who have school-age children at home. If you are in this situation, you are not alone. In the United States, around 20 percent of adults diagnosed with cancer have a child under eighteen.[1] Coping with cancer is hard for anyone. Having a child at home can bring an added layer of stress to a family. It can heighten both the practical and emotional challenges of cancer.

---

1. "Parents with Cancer: Tips for Talking to Kids," American Academy of Child and Adolescent Psychiatry, May 2019, www.aacap.org/AACAP/Families_and_Youth/Facts_for_Families/FFF -Guide/When-a-Parent-Has-Cancer-Tips-for-Talking-to-Kids-117.aspx.

YOUR CHILD IS UNIQUE

As we explore this topic, let's take a moment to recognize that every child is unique. Children are individuals with their own personalities and preferences. Your child will process the news of cancer in their own way. Age is a factor too. Children of different ages understand and approach information differently. It is important to share information with your child in an age-appropriate way. In this chapter, we highlight content from the Cancer Support Community's *What Do I Tell the Kids?* booklet. It touches on what children of various ages can understand and what they might be feeling.

TALKING WITH YOUR KIDS

Children, especially younger children, may hold certain myths and misconceptions about cancer that are important to acknowledge and address. For example, a child may think they did something to cause the cancer—like being disrespectful or defiant with a parent. Or they may fear that cancer is contagious, like the flu or a cold. They may also think that everyone who has cancer dies from it, especially if someone else you know has died from cancer.

This is why it is important to talk with your kids. They need to hear from you about what's going on and how it will affect them. You may want to protect them from the news, but children are smarter and more intuitive than we give them credit for. Your children may overhear conversations around the house or phone calls with doctors or friends. They may sense that something has changed. In the absence of information, they will draw their own conclusions.

Talking openly about cancer and acknowledging that this will be a challenging and sometimes scary time gives kids permission to cry or be angry, sad, or upset. Let your children know that you will answer any questions they have. They may feel awkward or hesitant at first, and that's okay, too. Meet them where they are. Open communication is key.

As you start to talk with your kids, try to prepare in advance for these conversations, especially the first conversation. Come with simply stated facts about your diagnosis and treatment plan. Focus on how this will affect them. Think of some honest but reassuring words to use. Tell them that you love them. Try to remember some key messages:

- Cancer is not their fault.
- Cancer is not contagious.
- Any question is okay.

Discuss the potential changes in your appearance so your children will not be caught off guard. Your hair loss, scarring, or weight loss could be traumatic for a child. Knowing what to expect in advance might ease their distress. You can even involve them in planning for those changes by taking them with you to the salon or barbershop if you plan to cut your hair short or shave your head, or having them help you pick out headscarves, turbans, or hats.

---

*"The conversation has to be all about them. Don't over-worry.
It doesn't have to be a long conversation. It should be very concrete and
address how their lives might change."*
—Sarah, metastatic breast cancer survivor

Here is some information about what children of different ages understand.[2] Try to tailor your conversations in an age-appropriate way.

---

2. Cancer Support Community, *Frankly Speaking About Cancer: What Do I Tell the Kids?*, 2014, www.cancersupportcommunity.org/sites/default/files/uploads/living-with-cancer/topics/guide/fsac_what_do_i_tell_the_kids.pdf.

Infancy to Toddlerhood (0 to 2 years)

WHAT CHILDREN UNDERSTAND

No understanding of cancer

Able to sense changes in day-to-day routines

Aware of changes in behavior and feelings of those around them

COMMON BEHAVIORS AND FEELINGS

More tantrums than usual

Changes in eating and sleeping habits

Separation anxiety—Difficulty separating from parents/caregivers (clingy)

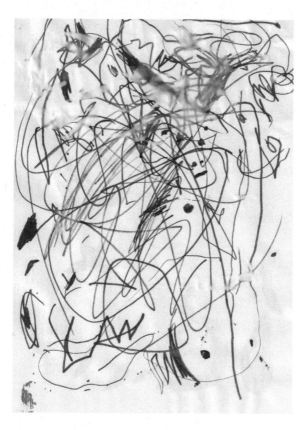

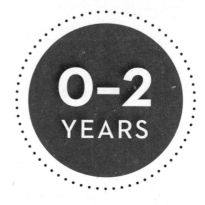

Preschool (3 to 5 years)

WHAT CHILDREN UNDERSTAND

Generally have some understanding of a simple illness like a cold but may not have any experience with, or understanding of, a serious illness like cancer

....

"Magical thinking"—Thinking they did something to cause cancer (e.g., "I wouldn't go to sleep and kept Mommy awake. She was very tired and I think I made her sick.")

COMMON BEHAVIORS AND FEELINGS

Regression—Acting younger than they are (e.g., suddenly wetting the bed even if they have been potty trained)

....

Short and intense bursts of emotion

....

Asking the same questions about cancer over and over again

....

Separation anxiety—Difficulty separating from parents/caregivers (clingy)

....

Playing or acting out themes related to doctors, sickness, and so on

3–5 YEARS

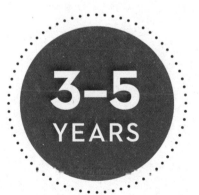

School Age (6 to 8 years)

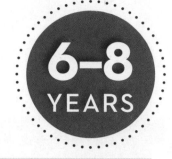

6–8 YEARS

WHAT CHILDREN UNDERSTAND

Can usually understand there is a difference between a simple illness (e.g., a cold) and a serious illness (e.g., cancer) but may not have had any experience with cancer

....

May have misinformation about cancer (e.g., may think cancer is contagious)

....

"Magical thinking"—Thinking they did something to cause cancer (e.g., "I wasn't behaving, and when Mommy told me to stop, I yelled at her and said some really mean things. I think I might have made Mommy sick.")

COMMON BEHAVIORS AND FEELINGS

Regression—Acting younger than they are (e.g., baby talk or wetting the bed)

....

Worrying about the person living with cancer as well as others (fear that others will become sick)

....

Asking questions related to physical changes (e.g., hair loss, bandages)

....

Showing anger if normal day-to-day routine is changed because of cancer (e.g., if they can't go to soccer practice because Dad is too sick to drive)

....

Separation anxiety—Difficulty separating from parents/caregivers (clingy)

....

Playing or acting out themes related to doctors, sickness, and so on

....

Distancing themselves from the sick parent because of fear or discomfort

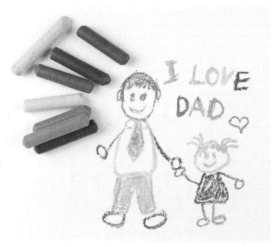

Preteen (9 to 12 years)

WHAT CHILDREN UNDERSTAND

Often have a basic understanding of cancer (have usually heard of cancer and even know of someone who has had cancer)

May have misinformation about cancer (e.g., may think cancer is contagious or that everyone who has cancer dies)

"Magical thinking"—Thinking they did something to cause cancer (e.g., "I haven't been doing well in school and my teachers have been calling home a lot. It's been making Mom upset and I think all the stress made her sick.")

COMMON BEHAVIORS AND FEELINGS

Showing anger if normal day-to-day routine is changed because of cancer (e.g., if they can't go to soccer practice because Dad is too sick to drive)

Hiding feelings from family and friends

Worrying that others will become sick

Showing fear and sadness as anger, and often directing it at family members

Feeling embarrassed by the sick parent because they are different

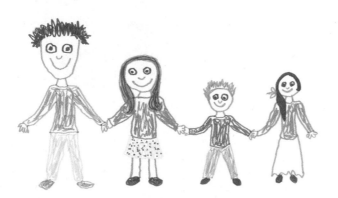

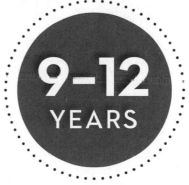

9–12 YEARS

Teens (13 to 18 years)

WHAT CHILDREN UNDERSTAND

Likely to have a basic understanding of what cancer is; able to understand many of the medical aspects of cancer

May have misinformation about cancer (e.g., may think cancer is contagious)

May be thinking more about life and death and the meaning of life

COMMON BEHAVIORS AND FEELINGS

Struggling between remaining close to family and trying to gain independence as a teenager

Showing anger if normal day-to-day routine is changed because of cancer (e.g., if they can't go to soccer practice because Dad is too sick to drive)

May not share feelings or talk openly with family or friends about the cancer experience

Taking out frustrations or anger on family members

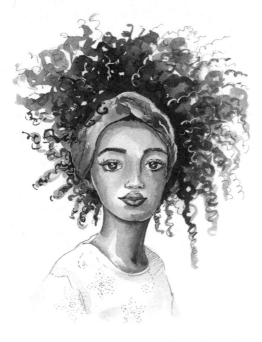

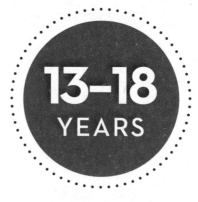

13–18 YEARS

PARENTING WITH CANCER

As you start treatment, also consider your child's life. Think about how to maintain and make the most of:

- *Routine:* Most children thrive on routine. Try to keep their routine and schedule as normal as possible. This applies to school, homework, mealtime, bedtime, or extracurricular activities. Routine gives children a sense of comfort and predictability, which they will welcome at a time when life may feel out of control.
- *Consistency:* Continue to enforce rules during this time. Make sure that kids keep up with chores and other responsibilities, like helping with younger siblings and completing homework. Look for ways to involve children in household activities, such as cooking and cleaning. By sharing the work, your children will feel empowered, like they are a part of the team contributing to your care and well-being. This can help build stronger family bonds and aid in the road to recovery.
- *Community:* You don't have to do this alone. Friends and family can help with rides, meals, and other tasks. In chapter nineteen, we will discuss digital tools, communities, and calendars to engage and organize your network. Consider sharing your cancer diagnosis with your child's teachers, school counselors, camp counselors, coaches, or other adults in their lives. These people can keep an eye out for any changes in behavior, attitude, or social interaction.

WHEN TO WORRY

As you go forward, you may notice changes in your child's behavior beyond what might be expected. Your child may be very clingy, anxious, upset, or angry. You might also observe changes in their eating or sleeping habits, or ability to focus or concentrate. If you are concerned, try to find support for them, the same way you would for yourself or your caregiver. Support may come from a social worker, therapist, or support group. Tweens and teens may benefit from an online community. There are also special camps for children whose parents have cancer. If you decide to try a private therapist, ask for a referral from your child's school or pediatrician—or from your primary care doctor. Be sure to check with your insurance company to see if it will pay for private sessions and, if so, how many.

YOU'RE IN THIS TOGETHER

As a parent, you have your children's needs and well-being foremost in your mind. Cancer brings uncertainty and stress into the home. It can disrupt the family dynamic. Yet it can also create an opportunity to strengthen family ties and bring a family closer together. By communicating openly and being transparent and honest with your children about what is happening, you will ensure that they feel included and comforted during this challenging time.

RESOURCES FOR TALKING WITH CHILDREN ABOUT CANCER

Camp Kesem—Free camp for children and teens whose parents have cancer. www .CampKesem.org

Cancer Support Community's "Talking to Kids and Teens About Cancer"—Resources and support to help talk with and support your children in the face of cancer. www .cancersupportcommunity.org/talking-kids-teens-about-cancer

Children's Treehouse—Support for children who are coping with a parent's or grandparent's cancer. www.ChildrensTreehousefdn.org

Jack and Jill Late Stage Cancer Foundation—WOW! Experiences for families facing late stage cancer. https://www.jajf.org

Marjorie E. Korff PACT (Parenting at a Challenging Time) Program—Resources and support for parents with cancer from Massachusetts General Hospital. www .mghpact.org

CHAPTER 18

Find Emotional Support

Cancer doesn't affect just our physical health. If you have cancer or are caring for someone with cancer, you also may begin to notice changes to your mental and emotional well-being. This is normal. Cancer can unleash a flood of emotions, from fear and anxiety to depression, anger, and deep sadness. Many people with cancer and their caregivers experience these feelings. You may mourn the loss of your life before cancer or worry about what life will look like after cancer. You may be concerned about your family and children or feel guilty that you can't care for them like you used to. You may fear that you will be in pain or that you may die from the disease.

Cancer is life altering. It brings changes you might not expect or might not be used to dealing with.

As you go forward, remember that you do not have to face cancer alone. There are support groups, counselors, social workers, telephone helplines, and online forums where you can share your concerns and get help. Support groups offer both counseling and community. But groups are not for everyone. Some people turn to friends, family, or a faith community. Or you may prefer private, one-on-one counseling. If so, ask your health care team for a referral. Look for a counselor or therapist who has experience with cancer. They will understand what you are going through. And check with your insurance provider to make sure they will cover private sessions, and if so, how many.

———

"Acknowledge the fear but take a step toward treatment. If you feel alone or you are alone, call a support person. Being alone is a choice. There is a support community available."
—Felicia, metastatic breast cancer survivor

———

QUESTIONS TO ASK YOURSELF WHEN SEEKING SUPPORT[1]

- What type of help do I want? (Help at home? Help with driving? Help with insurance?)
- Whom would I like to talk with about my next steps? Or join me at medical appointments?
- Who can help with practical support, such as work leave, family care, insurance, or driving?
- Can a website scheduler (like MyLifeLine) make it easy for friends and family to schedule times to help me?
- Can a cancer support organization provide me with useful services or information?
- Do I want to join a support group?

———

1. Cancer Support Community, *Frankly Speaking About Cancer: Multiple Myeloma*, February 2019, www.cancersupportcommunity.org/multiple-myeloma.

In chapter ten, we talked about distress screening. Some people feel overwhelmed with emotions when they are diagnosed with cancer, but they can't express the exact source of the distress. Distress screening is an effective tool to identify more specifically what concerns you. Be sure to ask a doctor, nurse, or social worker at your hospital or clinic to be screened for distress. When you do, also ask if there is a social worker or counselor on staff you can talk with.

"Get involved in a Cancer Support Community support group because they are not sad groups. People think we sit and cry. We don't. We laugh. We share knowledge. It's a great source of information."

—Diane, chronic myeloid leukemia survivor

In this chapter, we include some information from our *Frankly Speaking* series on how to cope with the emotional side of cancer. Part of coping is confronting your feelings. Once you do that, you can start to find the tools and resources to help you manage. You may be tempted to play down or ignore your distress or use drugs or alcohol to numb the pain. This inevitably backfires in the end.

Avoiding or suppressing strong feelings will only cause them to build up and come out in other ways. You may find yourself lashing out at friends, being irritable with your family, or withdrawing completely. By addressing your mental health needs, you not only will feel better emotionally but will be better able to focus on your physical health. Your stress level will be lower, and you may find a sense of balance. Research shows that engaging in healthy behaviors can help boost the immune system and improve our ability to fight disease.

FEELING LONELY OR ISOLATED[2]

People who lack a support network often feel lonely or isolated. This can increase their risk of depression or stress-related illnesses like heart disease. Some feelings of loneliness

---

2. Adapted from Cancer Support Community, *Frankly Speaking About Cancer: Feeling Isolated or Lonely*, April 2020, www.cancersupportcommunity.org/managing-stress-cancer.

are a normal reaction to a serious illness. These feelings may go away as you begin to feel better. When these feelings are extreme or long-lasting, they can lead to depression. Isolation and loneliness can also interfere with treatment. You may find it harder to participate actively in treatment, which may affect the outcome. If you are concerned that you do not have the social and emotional supports to help you through cancer, talk to your doctor, nurse, or social worker.

What You Can Do to Manage Feeling Lonely or Isolated

- Find someone to talk to about feeling lonely, such as family, friends, or your doctor, nurse, or social worker.
- Let your doctor, nurse, or social worker know if you do not feel you have a support system to help you at home or throughout your treatment and recovery. There are many community programs that can assist you with practical concerns. They can also help you feel less isolated at such a difficult time in your life.
- Join a support group or reach out to others in person, online, or by phone. Your social worker or nurse may have some suggestions about these services.
- Seek professional help. Try to find a therapist experienced in working with cancer patients. There is nothing shameful about receiving professional counseling. Thousands of people with cancer participate in individual, group, or family counseling. They find it to be very helpful in reducing the stress that cancer brings into their lives.

FEELING NERVOUS OR AFRAID[3]

If you feel nervous and afraid in a way that affects your ability to enjoy life, ask your doctor, nurse, or social worker for help. It is normal to feel some fear and anxiety when you have a serious illness. These feelings may go away as you begin to feel better. When these feelings

---

3. Adapted from Cancer Support Community, *Frankly Speaking About Cancer: Feeling Nervous or Afraid*, April 2020, www.cancersupportcommunity.org/managing-stress-cancer.

are extreme or long-lasting, they can lead to a more serious anxiety disorder. They can affect your ability to participate actively in your treatment and may even affect the outcome.

Symptoms That May Indicate You Need Help with Feeling Nervous or Afraid

- Feeling worried all the time
- Not being able to focus
- Not being able to "turn off thoughts" most of the time
- Trouble sleeping most nights
- Frequent crying spells
- Feeling afraid most of the time
- Having symptoms such as fast heartbeat, dry mouth, shaky hands, restlessness, or feeling on edge
- Anxiety that is not relieved by the usual ways to lessen anxiety, such as staying busy

FEELING SAD OR DEPRESSED[4]

Overwhelming sadness or depression can affect your ability to carry out daily activities and to participate actively in your treatment. It can also make physical symptoms more severe or have an impact on the treatment outcome. Know that you are not alone. It is important to talk about feeling sad or depressed with a family member, friend, clergy, or health care professional.

Signs and Symptoms of Depression

- Ongoing sad, anxious, or empty feelings
- Feeling hopeless or feeling guilty, worthless, or helpless
- Feeling irritable or restless

---

4. Adapted from Cancer Support Community, *Frankly Speaking About Cancer: Feeling Sad or Depressed*, April 2020, www.cancersupportcommunity.org/managing-stress-cancer.

- Loss of interest in activities or hobbies once enjoyable, including sex
- Feeling tired all the time
- Difficulty concentrating, remembering details, or making decisions
- Difficulty falling asleep or staying asleep, or sleeping all the time
- Overeating or loss of appetite
- Thoughts of death and suicide, or suicide attempts
- Ongoing aches and pains, headaches, cramps, or digestive problems that do not ease with treatment

WORRY ABOUT THE FUTURE[5]

People touched by cancer often experience three feelings: loss of control, unwanted aloneness, and loss of hope. These feelings can lead to worry about the future and uncertainty about what may lie ahead. This is a normal reaction. It becomes a problem only if you are so overcome with worry that you are unable to enjoy things that usually bring you pleasure.

If you find that you are extremely anxious about the future, reach out to a trusted friend, clergyperson, or mental health professional. Talk to your doctor, nurse, or social worker about your concerns. Some fears and concerns may be unfounded. They can be cleared up through a better understanding of cancer and your treatment plan. Your doctor may be able to prescribe medicine to reduce the stress and anxiety you are feeling.

Above all, know that it is a good idea to make plans for the future. Keep moving ahead one step at a time. It is okay to feel overwhelmed at times. Even before you had cancer, you might have had worries about your future.

Cancer can make some people feel like they've lost control of their body and their life. Having questions about the meaning of one's life is also normal. As you think, you may discover new goals, priorities, and possibilities. People with cancer often find that this chance to focus on what really matters can change the quality of their lives in positive ways. Having cancer can help you reconnect with the ways your life matters to you and make the changes that are important to you.

---

5. Adapted from Cancer Support Community, *Frankly Speaking About Cancer: Worry About the Future*, April 2020, www.cancersupportcommunity.org/managing-stress-cancer.

Many people focus on spending more time with family and friends. Others use this chance to complete a project such as a scrapbook or video. Still others decide to act on something they have always wanted to do, such as take up a new hobby or travel. There is no right answer that will work for all people. For each individual, the changes made or even the decision not to make any changes will be personal.

"You've got to have somebody to talk to. When something is bothering me, the support group is there."
—Steve, chronic lymphocytic leukemia survivor

You may find that, even after trying the ideas suggested here, you still feel depressed, anxious, or overwhelmed. In this case, it may be time to talk to your doctor about medicine to manage these symptoms. Antidepressant and antianxiety drugs can offer short-term relief during a stressful time. They can be another tool to help you approach cancer in a comprehensive way. Be sure to talk to your health care team about any drugs you are taking or considering taking. Some may interfere with cancer treatment.

While cancer can be hard emotionally, it can also lead to meaningful contemplation. You may reconsider your values and priorities. Use this time for self-reflection. Consider the things that really matter to you. How do you find meaning in this experience? How do you use it to turn a corner? Some people say that cancer made them realize they were in a bad job or an unhealthy relationship. For others, cancer offers an opportunity to heal old wounds. Still others say that cancer prompted them to finally take that dream trip or make more time for family. The cliché "stop and smell the roses" rings true for many people affected by cancer. Finding meaning in life with cancer can bring you joy, comfort, and gratification.

"Cancer has really shown me what's important and that's relationships with family and friends. Everything else is ancillary."
—Pete, acute myeloid leukemia survivor

You may feel that, when treatment ends, you should be back to normal and easily put everything behind you. Be patient with yourself. For many people, the emotional toll of cancer hits only after they put their energy into managing decisions, treatment, side effects, medical appointments, and finances. In chapter twenty-six, we will talk more about survivorship and what to expect post-treatment, but know that emotions and anxiety can bubble up at any time. Take those feelings seriously and seek support, no matter where you are on the cancer continuum. Help is out there.

ASK FOR HELP IF YOU NEED IT

If you find that feelings of loneliness, isolation, and despair continue to mount and you are having thoughts of harming yourself, pick up the phone and call 911 or go to the nearest emergency room. Or call the National Suicide Prevention Hotline, 800-SUICIDE (800-784-2433), to be connected to a suicide prevention center.

ACTIVE WAYS TO COPE[6]

- Take action to get rid of the problem.
- Plan how to deal with the problem.
- Look for advice and information to deal with the problem.
- Look for a sympathetic ear and emotional support.
- Accept that the problem exists and decide what you can and cannot control.
- Try to get a new perspective by making the best of the situation.
- Become aware of your feelings about the problem and express them to others.

6. Cancer Support Community, *Cancer Transitions: Moving Beyond Treatment Participant Workbook*, 2017, www.cancersupportcommunity.org/cancer-transitions.

RESOURCES FOR FINDING EMOTIONAL SUPPORT

Cancer Support Community's "Caregivers"—Cancer topics examined from the perspective of the caregiver. www.cancersupportcommunity.org/caregivers

Cancer Support Community's "Managing Stress from Cancer"—Resources on general coping and more specific concerns. www.cancersupportcommunity.org/managing-stress-cancer

Cancer Support Helpline—A free resource for people with cancer and their loved ones. Call with any question. 888-793-9355 or www.cancersupportcommunity.org/cancer-support-helpline

CHAPTER 19

Build Your Digital Support Network

We are living in the digital age. Technology is everywhere. We use apps to order food, catch a ride, book planes and trains, find babysitters, and track our steps. Our smartphones, tablets, and laptops are always nearby, at the ready, for whatever question or need arises. And, increasingly, technology is how we connect with each other and build community.

We have witnessed an explosion of online resources for people with cancer. From support groups to exercise classes to bulletin boards and listserves, the internet puts the world at our fingertips. Websites and apps help us learn about treatments, find doctors and clinical trials, and meet others with the same type of cancer. The opportunities are endless.

As you launch into cyberspace for information and support, proceed with caution. Research the online communities you use. Make sure they are private and transparent. Consider the tips in the following internet safety checklist.

INTERNET SAFETY CHECKLIST

- ❑   Know where you are. Who is hosting the online group or discussion board? Look for trusted sources like your hospital, the National Cancer Institute, or nonprofit organizations that you rely on. Most websites have an "About" section. Go there to learn more about a new site before you start using their resources or commenting on their boards.

- ❑   See if the site is password protected. Can you set and change your password?

- ❑   Check out the privacy policy of the site. Is the site private? Are the discussions confidential? Who can read your comments? Some websites and online groups allow you to use a "username." A handle is an anonymous name that you use online so you don't have to use your real name. It helps protect your privacy. Have fun coming up with a creative handle that reflects your personality or interests.

- ❑   Avoid joining a site where the user list is sold or shared. Investigate whether the website sells its information or trades user lists with other groups or businesses.

- ❑   Check out policies around solicitation. Once you join a site, will you and your network be bombarded with requests for donations? Will there be ads asking you to buy things or spend money in other ways? Avoid websites that require you to enter a credit card before using their resources.

- ❑   Look for oversight. See if the discussion or forum is monitored by a professional, such as a nurse, doctor, or social worker. This person plays a critical role. They can remove misinformation and inappropriate content.

At the Cancer Support Community, we host an online community called MyLife-Line. Here, patients and families can set up their own personal websites, learn about cancer, connect with others facing cancer, and share their experiences. Below are some of the features you can find at MyLifeLine:

Personal website: You can set up your own personal, private site where invited friends and family members can follow your progress and read your updates. Patients and caregivers often tell us it is overwhelming, even stressful, to try to keep everyone up-to-date on what is happening. Some people even feel guilty because they can't reply to everyone or return all the emails, texts, and calls. By setting up a personal site on MyLifeLine or through another platform (some are listed below), you can keep everyone informed. You decide what you feel comfortable sharing. You can add pictures, videos, stories, or poems and invite others to do the same. You can even ask a friend or family member to help maintain and update the site.

Helping calendar: The helping calendar is a tool to organize your social network. It allows you and your family to request assistance with specific tasks. Your friends are able to offer help without duplicating efforts. Use it to coordinate meals, request rides for kids, find someone to walk the dog, or ask a friend to accompany you to a medical appointment or go on a walk with you. You can also use it to keep track of your treatment schedule. It's simple to use. You post a list of tasks or needs on the calendar and the folks you invite can sign up for one or more. Most people find that friends, coworkers, and neighbors want to help. An online tool like this helping calendar gives them an easy, efficient way to do so.

Discussion boards: Discussion boards are online forums where patients and caregivers connect around a specific topic. It may be a cancer type or other area of shared interest like living with breast cancer, nutrition and wellness, parenting with cancer, or survivorship. The boards are monitored by a social worker and allow people to ask questions and share tips and feelings. They can be a good way to meet other people who are having the same experience.

"When my husband was diagnosed, I wanted to stay in touch with others but didn't have a lot of time, so I used MyLifeLine. I posted every couple of days and I got so much in return. For example, I would ask, 'Could somebody help me with research?' I'd get lots of answers. My community even set up this caravan of dinners. This gave me the love and support that I needed to stay strong."
—Candice, caregiver of loved one with cancer

The internet can be a lifeline for people with cancer. Virtual communities and online groups provide inspiration and connection both to others with cancer and to your own network of loved ones. They can offer a comfortable space where you can express your feelings and emotions, and an easy way to keep friends and family updated on your journey. Ask questions and use the tips in this chapter to find a safe and welcoming online community to support you through treatment and beyond.

DIGITAL RESOURCES TO SEEK AND ORGANIZE SUPPORT

Cancer.Net Mobile: The American Society of Clinical Oncology site provides a place to save information about prescription medications, a symptom tracker, and an interactive tool to keep track of questions to ask your health care provider and record their voice answers. www.cancer.net/navigating-cancer-care/managing-your-care/cancer net-mobile

Meal Train—Organize meals or other activities for a friend or loved one. mealtrain.com

MyLifeLine—The Cancer Support Community can help you organize information and keep friends and loved ones updated. www.cancersupportcommunity.org/mylifeline

CHAPTER 20

Focus on Nutrition

When you have cancer, parts of your life can feel beyond your control. One of the ways to regain control is to focus on your everyday health. Nutrition can be key to this. Eating healthy foods can give you strength, boost your energy, and even help with side effects.

Cancer treatment can bring side effects that have an impact on what you eat. You may notice nausea, diarrhea, constipation, weight loss, mouth sores, or loss of appetite. Your taste for certain foods may change. Our emotional state can also affect what we eat and how our bodies process food, so refer to chapter eighteen for tools to help you cope with the emotions of cancer.

Understanding your body's food and dietary needs and addressing them can help you feel empowered and in control. It is another way in which you can be an active member of your own health care team. Some people use a cancer diagnosis as a catalyst for lifestyle change for themselves *and* their partner or family. Learning more about vegetables, grains, proteins, and healthy eating trends can become a family activity. Children who love superheroes might get excited about the idea of superfoods.

One of the first steps is to get professional help with nutrition. Try these sources for guidance on food and nutrition:

Hospital dietician: More and more hospitals are hiring registered dieticians to support patients' nutritional needs. A registered dietician (RD) has training in diet, nutrition, and food. If they have "CSO" after their name, they are a board-certified specialist in oncology nutrition. This certification focuses on the unique nutritional needs of people with cancer. If there is not an RD at the hospital, ask your health care team to refer you to someone in your community. Remember to check to see if your insurance will cover a dietician visit. Some do; some do not.

Trusted resources: Ask your health care team for advice. They can provide the names of organizations that can help with eating tips, recipes, and more. Also, use the free resources on diet and nutrition listed at the end of this chapter.

As you start to focus on your diet, be mindful of:

- *Food safety.* Cancer treatment can weaken your immune system, so it is extra important to pay attention to food safety. Remember to:
  - keep cooking and kitchen surfaces clean.
  - keep foods at the proper temperature.
  - avoid uncooked or raw foods like sushi and undercooked meats, and unpasteurized foods like some milks and cheeses.
- *Help that may harm.* Many people take vitamins and other supplements for nutrition. Discuss all pills or herbs you are taking or plan to take with your health care team. Some may interfere with your treatment. Talk to your doctor if you plan to start a specific diet, especially one that emphasizes certain foods or types of foods. You do not know how your body will react to drastic changes.

You may have noticed a pullout section in this book with tasty, nutritious recipes. The Cancer Support Community created these recipes in partnership with the American Institute for Cancer Research (AICR). AICR's mission is to "champion research that increases understanding of the relationship between nutrition, lifestyle, and cancer." These recipes were developed by a registered dietician and certified specialist in cancer nutrition, with oversight by a medical advisory board.

HELPFUL TIPS TO MANAGE YOUR NUTRITION[1]

These tips can help with healthy eating during cancer treatment:

- When you just don't feel like eating, consider drinking a liquid or powdered meal replacement (such as "instant breakfast").
- Consider eating five or six small meals each day instead of three large meals.
- You may find it helps to eat smaller amounts at any one time. This can keep you from feeling too full and may help reduce nausea.
- Keep snacks nearby for when you feel like eating. Take easy-to-carry snacks such as peanut butter crackers, nuts, granola bars, or dried fruit when you go out.
- Find ways to add extra protein and healthy calories to your diet.
- Drink liquids throughout the day—even when you do not want to eat. Choose liquids that add calories and other nutrients such as juice, soup, milk, and soy-based drinks with protein.
- Try eating a light bedtime snack. This will give extra calories but won't affect your appetite for the next meal.
- Change the form of a food. For instance, you might make a fruit milkshake or smoothie instead of eating a piece of fruit.
- Eat soft, cool, or frozen foods. These include ice cream, yogurt, milkshakes, and popsicles.
- Eat larger meals when you feel well and are rested. For many people, this is in the morning after a good night's sleep.
- Sip only small amounts of liquids during meals. Many people feel too full if they eat and drink at the same time. If you want more than just small sips, have a larger drink at least thirty minutes before or after meals.

---

1. Cancer Support Community, *Frankly Speaking About Cancer: Eating and Nutrition*, April 2020, www.cancersupportcommunity.org/diet-nutrition.

KEEP A FOOD DIARY

Sometimes it is difficult to know how specific foods will affect you throughout the day, or even remember what you had for breakfast! This diary can
help you keep track of what you are eating and how you feel.[2] Make copies
of this page to keep in a binder or folder.

Daily Food & Symptoms Diary   Date: _____

Make copies of this and fill out daily.

Breakfast			Time:
Food & Drinks	Serving Size	Symptoms	
			❏ Mild ❏ Moderate ❏ Severe

Lunch			Time:
Food & Drinks	Serving Size	Symptoms	
			❏ Mild ❏ Moderate ❏ Severe

---

2. Cancer Support Community, *Frankly Speaking About Cancer: Eating Well During Cancer Treatment*, December 2018, www.cancersupportcommunity.org /diet-nutrition.

Dinner			Time:	
Food & Drinks	Serving Size	Symptoms		
			❑ Mild	
			❑ Moderate	
			❑ Severe	

Snacks			Time:	
Food & Drinks	Serving Size	Symptoms		
			❑ Mild	
			❑ Moderate	
			❑ Severe	

Did you make any changes to your eating habits today? If yes, what did you change? Did it help any symptoms?

_____

_____

_____

_____

_____

_____

_____

_____

_____

_____

_____

_____

Let's address specific side effects. Use these concrete tips to help manage them and feel better:[3]

Constipation

Food Tips for Constipation

- Increase intake of foods that can help promote a bowel movement:
    - Choose high-fiber foods, such as whole grains, fruits, vegetables, nuts, and beans.
    - Try prunes and other dried fruits and juices, such as prune or apple juice.
    - Drink hot beverages, such as herbal tea and decaffeinated coffee.
- Make sure you drink enough fluids.
- If you are having gas and bloating, stay away from "gassy" vegetables like cabbage, broccoli, cauliflower, peas, corn, and beans. Avoid drinking through a straw or chewing gum. These can also make gas and bloating worse.

Other Tips for Constipation

- Move more if you are able—walk, stretch, or do yoga.
- Talk to your health care team about drugs or other tips that can help with constipation.

Diarrhea

Foods to Avoid When You Have Diarrhea

- Alcohol and caffeinated drinks
- Dairy foods (other than cultured dairy like yogurt or kefir)
- Foods that are high in sugar, such as juices or sweets
- Greasy and fried foods
- High-fiber and bulky foods, such as raw vegetables, nuts, and whole grains

---

3. Cancer Support Community, *Frankly Speaking: Eating Well During Cancer Treatment.*

Easy-to-Digest Foods to Eat When You Have Diarrhea

- Apples (without skin) or applesauce
- Baked chicken, turkey, or fish
- Bananas
- Canned fruit (in juice), such as canned peaches or pears
- Oatmeal, barley, or cream of rice cereal
- Plain potatoes without skin
- White rice or pasta

Other Tips for Diarrhea

- Drink hydrating fluids with electrolytes, such as coconut water, broth, electrolyte drinks, and diluted fruit juices. Carry a water bottle to stay hydrated.
- Get probiotics by eating foods such as yogurt, kefir, and fermented foods. Talk to your health care team before taking any probiotic supplement.

Dry Mouth

Food Tips for Dry Mouth

- Avoid alcohol and limit caffeinated drinks.
- Increase your saliva by:
  - sucking on sugar-free tart candies prior to eating.
  - chewing on sugar-free gum in between meals.
  - moistening foods with sauces and gravies.
- If acidic foods don't irritate your mouth or throat, you can also try:
  - adding lemon or lime to water.
  - using citrus fruits or juices in marinades or dressings.
- Limit dry or hard-to-swallow foods, such as baked potatoes, peanut butter, tough meat, and "doughy" bread.
- Make sure you drink enough fluids to prevent dehydration. Carry a water bottle with you to stay hydrated.

Other Tips for Dry Mouth

- Apply lip balm or petroleum jelly to protect your lips.
- Sleep with a humidifier in your room to help moisten your mouth at night. Be sure to clean the humidifier regularly.
- Use alcohol-free mouthwash daily and/or saliva substitutes.

Challenges with Preparing or Obtaining Healthy Food

Tips to Manage Fatigue and Prepare Healthy Food

- Ask family and friends to help make meals and assist with other daily tasks.
- On days when you have more energy, cook soup or stews in bulk to have meals on hand.
- Increase your physical activity as much as you can in order to help fight fatigue.
- Take it one day at a time and look at each day as a new day.
- Take breaks throughout the day.
- Try something you did not do yesterday and try not to let your lack of energy discourage you.
- Try not to overdo it on higher-energy days, so you can conserve your energy.

Tips to Obtain Healthy Food

- Finding healthy food can be difficult, which can be frustrating if you're trying to eat well. We understand that some communities lack stores that sell healthy foods. In some areas, it is possible to order groceries online to be delivered to your home. Ask your neighbors or health care team if they know of websites to try. Also, use the resources at the end of this chapter.
- Healthy food can be costly. Often, people want to eat healthy but find they cannot afford it. Use the resources at the end of this chapter to find free or low-cost food in your community. Also, let your health care team know that you need help with food. Many organizations will provide healthy foods to people who are older, sick, or unable to afford food.
- Even if you can afford food, you may be eligible to receive a food box for free or at a low cost due to age or having cancer.

Mouth Sores and Mouth Pain

Food Tips for Mouth Sores and Mouth Pain

- Choose foods that help soothe the mouth, including:
  - cold foods, such as popsicles, frozen fruit, and ice cream.
  - soft, mild foods, such as cottage cheese, smoothies, and yogurt.
  - well-cooked, soft meals such as potatoes, macaroni and cheese, casseroles, stews, and ground meats.
- Avoid foods that could irritate the mouth, including:
  - acidic or spicy foods, such as citrus fruits, tomatoes, peppers, and vinegar.
  - alcohol and carbonated drinks.
  - crunchy or hard foods, such as crusty bread, pretzels, and chips.
  - hot foods—choose room temperature or cold instead.

Other Tips for Mouth Sores and Mouth Pain

- Drink through a straw to avoid sore spots.
- Suck on ice chips when you have mouth pain.
- Use a baking soda rinse before and after meals.

Changes in Taste and Smell

If everything tastes bland or has no taste:

- Add stronger flavors to foods. Pickles, condiments, sauces, dressings, vinegar, or citrus juices may help. (You may need to avoid these if you have mouth or throat sores.)
- Add spices and seasonings to enhance the flavor of your foods.
- Marinate meats for a stronger flavor.
- Suck on sugar-free lemon or lime candies before or after a meal.
- Clean your mouth with a homemade baking soda rinse.

If everything tastes metallic or bitter:

- Add sweeteners such as honey or pure maple syrup to foods to offset the bitter taste.
- Choose other protein sources (such as fish, chicken, or beans) if red meat tastes metallic.
- Use plastic utensils instead of silverware.
- Avoid cooking on iron skillets.

If the smell of food makes you not want to eat:

- Avoid being in the kitchen when food is being made.
- Understand that foods may taste or smell different every day. You may find it helpful to keep trying different foods to find what appeals to you.
- Choose cold or room-temperature foods instead of hot foods, which can smell stronger.
- Light a scented candle or essential oil diffuser to remove unpleasant or offensive odors.
- Open a window or turn on a fan to minimize the smells.

Nausea and Vomiting

Food Tips for Nausea and/or Vomiting

- Even though you do not feel like eating, an empty stomach can make nausea worse. Aim to eat a small amount of food every one to two hours to prevent nausea.
- Choose bland foods, such as plain pasta or rice. If dry mouth isn't a problem, you can also try dry foods such as crackers and pretzels.
- Choose room-temperature or cold foods, instead of hot entrées.
- Drink ginger tea or chew ginger candies when you feel nauseous.
- Drink hydrating fluids (such as water, 100 percent juice, coconut water, or chamomile or ginger tea) throughout the day to prevent dehydration.
- Limit your intake of fried, greasy, or "heavy" foods, as these can make nausea worse.

Other Tips for Nausea and/or Vomiting

- If drugs or supplements make you nauseous, talk to your health care team about taking them with food, instead of on an empty stomach.
- Talk to your health care team about anti-nausea drugs. For the most benefit, take anti-nausea drugs thirty to forty minutes prior to a meal. You may also need to take them around the clock, instead of as needed.
- Try deep breathing, meditation, or guided imagery to help settle your stomach and mind.

RESOURCES FOR HEALTHY EATING

Academy of Nutrition and Dietetics—Click on "Find an Expert" and "Search by Expertise" to find a cancer/oncology nutrition dietitian. 800-877-1600 or www.eatright.org

American Institute for Cancer Research—Education, activities for adults and children, and resources related to cancer and nutrition. 800-843-8114 or www.aicr.org

Body and Soul: A Celebration of Healthy Eating and Living for African Americans—The National Cancer Institute's church-based outreach effort to promote healthy eating among African Americans. ebccp.cancercontrol.cancer.gov/programDetails.do?programId=257161

Cancer Support Community's "Diet and Nutrition"—A go-to resource for education, support, and recipes related to cancer and eating. www.cancersupportcommunity.org/diet-nutrition

Feeding America—Find your local food bank. www.feedingamerica.org

Foodpantries.org—Find free or reduced-cost food in your community. www.foodpantries.org

National Cancer Institute's *Eating Hints: Before, During, and After Cancer Treatment*. Free booklet including tips for eating well before, during, and after cancer treatment. 800-4-CANCER or www.cancer.gov/cancerinfo/eatinghints

Oldways—A food and nutrition nonprofit focused on healthy eating and cultural food traditions. 617-421-5500 or www.oldwayspt.org

CHAPTER 21

Exercise and Mind-Body Techniques

Like nutrition, which we discussed in chapter twenty, exercise and mind-body techniques can help you feel empowered and take back some control of your life in the face of cancer. You may not feel up to your old workout and wellness routines. This is understandable. A modified approach, which is adapted for you, can have physical and mental benefits. It can even help with healing and recovery.

"I wouldn't accept other people's perceptions of what a cancer patient should be or can do."
—Sarah, on starting CrossFit during treatment for metastatic breast cancer

------

EXERCISE

If you're someone who hasn't exercised much in life, you may be thinking that you're not going to start now. Before you stop here, take a minute to consider the many benefits of exercise. An exercise program that is tailored to your specific needs and abilities can help you:[1]

- keep or improve your physical abilities.
- improve your balance and lower your risk of falls or broken bones.
- lower your risk of heart disease and osteoporosis.
- improve your blood flow and lower your risk of blood clots.
- improve your self-esteem.
- improve your sexual functioning.
- lower your risk of anxiety and depression.
- reduce the impact of side effects such as nausea and fatigue.
- sleep better.
- reduce "chemo brain," for more clarity in learning and thinking.
- control your weight and prevent constipation.

Exercise can take on many forms—like walking, jogging, biking, lifting light weights, gentle stretching, swimming, and more. You may want to explore a few to find the right one for you. If you are someone who exercised before cancer, you may feel uncomfortable going to your usual gym or classes. If this is the case, look for wellness programs that are adapted specifically for people with cancer. They may be available through your hospital or cancer center, or at a community organization like the YMCA or local Cancer Support Community affiliate. You also may find instruction online.

Some people use their cancer diagnosis to discover new forms of exercise like yoga, tai chi, or qigong. What are these practices and how can they help?

---

1. Adapted from "Exercise for Wellness," Cancer Support Community, accessed November 12, 2020, www.cancersupportcommunity.org/living-cancer/exercise-wellness.

- *Yoga:* Yoga originated in India. It is a series of physical movements and meditations that can help with posture, strength, balance, and stress relief. Some cancer centers and community organizations have developed yoga classes just for people with cancer. Many cancer patients tell us they enjoy yoga because it helps with both physical and mental stress and enables them to find balance and relaxation.
- *Tai chi:* Tai chi is a Chinese martial arts practice. It is used to enhance focus, flexibility, and strength. It consists of a series of slow motions and deep breathing. Tai chi is known to help with balance and potentially reduce falls.
- *Qigong:* Qigong (also known as chi gung) is another ancient Chinese practice. It is designed to restore balance to one's qi (pronounced "chi"), which means life energy. It involves slow, gentle movements and deep breathing and may help with health and healing.

When starting to exercise, some people find it helpful to write out a plan, set goals, and track their progress. This chapter includes an exercise log that you can photocopy and keep in a binder. Consider keeping it with the Daily Food and Symptoms Diary provided in chapter twenty.

As you begin to exercise during and after treatment, take it slowly. It is important not to overdo it. Set realistic goals that align with how you are feeling. Start with a more modest program that will help you achieve your goals and feel good about your progress. For some, this may mean walking around the dining room table two or three times a day. For others, it could mean a walk outside or perhaps some gentle stretching or light weights. Talk with your health care team about your exercise program. Surgery and treatment may limit some of your physical abilities. You want to avoid causing any harm. Your team may be able to suggest exercises for you or refer you to a physical therapist or other expert in movement and recovery.

"Stay as positive as you can. Reach out to other people in the same circumstances. Try to stay active. It's hard to go to the store or just walk around the block when you don't feel well, but it's important to keep moving."

—Christine, tonsil cancer survivor

My Exercise Log

Goal for the Week:

Date	Type of Exercise/ Activity	Length of Time	Distance/ Steps	How did you feel before and after your exercise? Did you face any challenges?

MIND-BODY TECHNIQUES

Exercise is not the only way people with cancer manage stress and restore health and well-being. Mind-body techniques can help you center yourself, find meaning in the cancer experience, and reestablish a sense of calm and well-being. Many people with cancer benefit from meditation and guided imagery.

Meditation

Meditation allows you to focus your mind and remove distracting thoughts and other "clutter" for better mental clarity and emotional calm. It can help reduce stress, improve your attention span, and promote feelings of peace and tranquility. Meditation takes patience and practice; it is a skill you can develop and improve over time.

You may hear about different forms of meditation. One example is mindfulness meditation. According to Jon Kabat-Zinn:

> Mindfulness is the awareness that arises when we non-judgmentally pay attention in the present moment. It cultivates access to core aspects of our own minds and bodies that our very sanity depends on. Mindfulness, which includes tenderness and kindness, restores dimensions of our being. These have never actually been missing, just that we have been missing them, we have been absorbed elsewhere. When your mind clarifies and opens, your heart also clarifies and opens.[2]

Take time to explore different meditation techniques and see how they make you feel. Remember, the benefits won't happen overnight. Meditation is like strengthening and conditioning a muscle; it takes time, effort, and commitment.

---

2. Ed Shapiro and Deb Shapiro, *The Unexpected Power of Mindfulness and Meditation* (Mineola, NY: Ixia Press, 2019), 7.

Guided Imagery

Guided imagery is a relaxation technique in which you think of positive images to create a sense of calm and well-being. It is best to sit down or lie in a quiet, peaceful place when you practice this technique. Close your eyes, breathe deeply, and center yourself to prepare.

The guest essay by Maria Fanelli details an example guided imagery exercise you can use to practice. You can try this as written or insert your own imagery. The goal is to find a pathway that feels good to you—your "happy place."

"Gilda's Club has been wonderful. The meditation and mindfulness classes were very helpful. I learned different coping mechanisms. I am so thankful for Gilda's, especially because it's free to cancer patients."

—Laura, multiple myeloma survivor

Regardless of the approach you choose, focusing on moving or relaxing your body can help with fatigue, sleep issues, depression, balance, and other challenges you may face with, through, and beyond cancer. Find a program and routine that works for you. Set realistic goals. Perhaps invite a family member or friend to join you. Having a workout or meditation partner may help you keep your commitment to take care of yourself. Even a small level of activity can make a big difference in how you feel each day.

Guided Imagery Exercise

MARIA FANELLI, LLC

Maria Fanelli is a seasoned mindfulness instructor, life coach, and mind-body health educator who teaches clients how to clarify and cultivate a forward path to their goals.

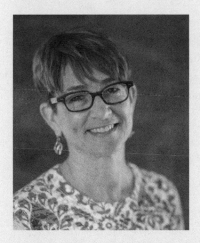

LOVE is a guided imagery and relaxation meditation to use during a cancer treatment. This is a meditation you can guide yourself through during any cancer treatment, and you can spend as little or as much time as you like with this exercise. The letters stand for:

L: Let go
O: Observe
V: Visualize
E: Energy

Let's begin! Settle comfortably into your spot—a posture where you feel relaxed, yet awake. Breathe in a somewhat deeper breath, if that is comfortable for you, and allow the breath to release on its own. Let's do it again, one more breath. Now you are ready!

L: LET GO—LETTING GO OF TENSION

Start by feeling into your body and notice where you feel any tension or energy . . . It is often helpful to do a quick scan of your body from the top of your head to your toes by "feeling" into each area. Whenever you notice any tightness, tension, or sensations of energy, take a deep breath and imagine the breath flowing into and out of that area. As you inhale, relax and allow the area to open or loosen. As you exhale, feel or imagine all the tension or tightness leaving—letting it go.

This is where scanning the body is often helpful. You may notice areas that are tight or tense that you were not previously aware of. With this exercise, when you notice tense or tight areas, you are going to allow relaxation to flow into those areas. Imagine your breath flowing out and spreading relaxation throughout your body. From your head to your toes, feel relaxation flowing and spreading throughout the entire body, causing all the muscles to relax and any tension to dissipate.

It's flowing down from the head, the face, if the jaw is held tightly perhaps allowing the jaw to drop ever so slightly . . . relaxation flowing into the neck and shoulders, allowing the shoulders to drop . . . feeling relaxation spreading to the arms, hands, and fingers, then flowing down the torso, the front and back of the torso, moving the attention to the stomach area and into the pelvis. Feeling relaxation in the buttocks and relaxation flowing into the legs and feet and toes.

Then feeling relaxation in the entire body.

O: OBSERVE—OBSERVING THE BREATH AND SENSATIONS

With an awareness of the entire body, observe the sensations of your body breathing. You are breathing normally. Now bring your full attention to actually feeling the breath flowing into and out of the body. Feel the full inhale from when it first begins and feel the full exhale all the way to the end before a new breath begins. Nice and easy. Breathing in, breathing out. Following the flow of the breath with your attention. You can use this breath as your center that you can always come back to.

Now, notice and observe any other sensations in the body. Be curious! Sometimes you may notice very subtle sensations in different areas of the body like warmth or coolness, tingling, vibrating, numbness, or perhaps not much at all. However, you are turning your attention away from anything that is currently happening outside the body to observing how the body is feeling inside. Use the breath to keep you relaxed and steady and just observe and notice any other sensations that are present. Notice the characteristics of each sensation and continue to feel relaxation all around the area of the sensations. Whatever the sensations feel like, acknowledge and welcome them. Allow them to be here—knowing they will continue to come and go and change all during your treatment. They are always changing. Allow them to come and go and change.

V: VISUALIZE—VISUALIZING HEALTH AND HAPPINESS

Continue to use the breath to keep you centered and welcome any sensations that are present. You can also continue to soften any noticeable tension. Now close your eyes and take yourself to your favorite place . . . It's a special place in your life. A place where you feel comfortable, relaxed, and happy. Put yourself in your favorite clothes and your favorite colors. The weather is perfect for you. Imagine doing all the things you love to do. Allow yourself to rest here in your place where you are happy, relaxed, and calm.

You may begin to notice the sounds around you in your special place. Feel how good you are feeling and how happy you are. Notice all the things you love that are present. Know that because you are feeling so relaxed and happy, your healthy cells are very receptive to your treatment. Imagine whatever treatment you are receiving making your cells healthy and rejuvenated. All your cells are responding well and they feel stronger and healthier than ever before. Your treatment is bringing health and happiness to all your cells and your body and your healthy cells continue to multiply as toxins and cancer cells continue to leave and dissolve.

E: ENERGY—ENERGIZING YOUR BODY

Feel your body receiving positive energy right now. It is flowing through your entire body. Imagine this positive energy flowing in through the top of your head in the form of a brilliant white light, and flowing down throughout your entire body. It is bringing health and positive energy to every area of your body. Feel this energetic, brilliant, powerful white light flowing down through the top of your head and filling your entire body with health and healing and pure energy. It even spreads outside your body. You can imagine the rays of the light glowing all around you, streaming out like the rays of the sun. This is healing energy that rejuvenates your body and soul and makes you feel so alive and empowered.

More empowered than you have felt in a long time. Even after your treatment today, you remember that this light energy will stay with you—bringing continued health, healing, and love.

Breathing in, breathing out . . .

Perhaps acknowledging that you took the time to care for yourself today during your treatment. Remember, you can always do a short version of the LOVE meditation anytime during the day—letting go of tension, observing sensations, visualizing health and happiness, and feeling healing energy flow through you—as you stay anchored on the breath.

RESOURCES FOR EXERCISE AND MIND-BODY TECHNIQUES

Cancer Support Community's "Exercise for Wellness"—Learn how to develop and maintain an exercise plan. www.cancersupportcommunity.org/living-cancer/exercise-wellness

Cancer Support Community's "Gentle Customized Exercise"—Exercises to get started. www.cancersupportcommunity.org/gentle-customized-exercise

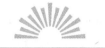

CHAPTER 22

Focus on Finances

It is very likely that cancer will have a financial impact on you and your family. You may have added medical costs like co-pays, deductibles, and other out-of-pocket expenses, all of which we discussed in chapter nine. Cancer can also result in lost wages or extra childcare, gas, or parking expenses. Whatever your financial situation, cancer will take a toll.

We often talk about the side effects of cancer treatment. Usually we mean the health-related side effects, like nausea, hair loss, and fatigue. Money problems can be another side effect of cancer. This is referred to as "financial toxicity." Financial toxicity can lead to mounting debt, often in the form of unpaid hospital bills or credit card bills. It can affect your health, too. As finances becomes tight, people with cancer sometimes skip medical appointments or drug doses to save money. This can have a lasting impact on treatment and recovery. Try to focus on your finances early on to prevent finding yourself in this situation. There are programs and services to help ease the financial burden of cancer. It may take a little time to find them. We encourage you to ask for help.

"When I was diagnosed with leukemia, I did not cry. But when I was told how much the medicine was going to cost, that's when I cried."
—Diane, chronic myeloid leukemia survivor

FIND HELP

As you build your cancer care team, see if there is a family member or trusted friend who can help with insurance, billing, and other financial matters. This person can find answers to questions and ensure that paperwork is done right away. By focusing on finances at the onset, you may reduce or prevent toxicity. You can also ask for help at your hospital or cancer center, or at a community organization. Many have social workers and financial counselors who can help with money questions, bills, and insurance matters. At the end of this book (see page 251), we list groups that can help with co-pay assistance and other out-of-pocket expenses.

"The cost for my treatment is particularly overwhelming. The prices are in the thousands and thousands of dollars, and nobody, even if you're wealthy, can afford that kind of money each month. So I am thankful for different charitable organizations that step up and help with that. Otherwise, I probably wouldn't be here because I couldn't take that medicine."
—Diane, chronic myeloid leukemia survivor

ASK QUESTIONS

People with cancer often say that finances are one of the most stressful parts of dealing with a cancer diagnosis. In the United States, our health care system adds to the challenge. Bills and payments come from different places, and it is hard to figure out how much services and medicines will cost. If you are buying a new car or a television, for example, you know the cost and you can comparison shop at different locations. This is not the case in health care. Two people with the exact same diagnosis treated at the same hospital could have very different co-pays and out-of-pocket costs, depending on their insurance plans. It is important to get as much information as possible up front about your diagnosis and the recommended treatment plan. Ask questions and try to learn as much as you can about costs in advance.

GET ORGANIZED

Here are a few tips to help you get organized around financial matters:

Practical Tips for Gathering Cost Information[1]

- Make sure that you and your providers submit any bills to your insurance company in a timely manner. Many insurance companies will not pay a claim submitted after the time period specified in the policy.
- Submit *all* medical expenses even if you are aren't sure whether they are covered. If you don't submit, the insurance company definitely won't pay!
- Review bills and keep accurate records of claims submitted, both pending and paid. This usually includes matching bills you receive from providers with explanations of benefits (EOBs) you receive from the insurance company.
- Keep copies of anything related to your claims. You can do this yourself, or you can ask a friend or family member (someone who is organized!) to help. Examples of items you should have on file include:
  - medical bills from all health care providers
  - claims filed
  - reimbursement or payment statements and EOBs received from insurance companies
  - dates, names, and outcomes of contacts made with insurers and others
  - nonreimbursed or outstanding medical and related costs
  - dates of admission to hospitals or other health care facilities, clinic visits, lab work, diagnostic tests, procedures, and treatments
  - records of medications received and prescriptions filled

---

1. Adapted from "Practical Tips for Gathering Cost Information," Cancer Support Community, accessed October 21, 2020, www.cancersupportcommunity.org/help-managing-cancer-costs.

- Get a notebook or accordion folder to organize paperwork and record all expenses, conversations with the insurance company, doctor's appointments, exams, and other pertinent information. Keep track of phone calls by noting the date and time of the call, the name of the person you spoke with, what they said, and their contact information.
- Pick a certain day of the week to be "health care bill day." Use this time to get organized, using the suggestions above. This will help you get the work done without feeling like it is taking over your everyday life.
- Identify an easily accessible place in your house that will not be disturbed by others where you can store your bills, paperwork, and files.

"The clinical trial picked up my co-pay so I wasn't out as much financially as I thought I would be. My social worker found a grant for me from Lazarex Cancer Foundation that would pay for my Ubers to the clinic. As long as I was in the clinical trial, they would pay for all my transportation."
—Wendy, breast cancer survivor

ADDITIONAL TIPS

If your insurance plan includes a deductible, you can expect to have higher out-of-pocket costs for the first two to three months after your diagnosis. The higher the deductible, the longer it may take to reach that threshold. Also, insurance tends to reset in the new year. You may have higher costs starting again in January.

We know that it can be difficult to talk about money. You may be uncomfortable asking for help. It may be reassuring to know that you are not alone. Many, if not most, people with cancer have told us that money worries have been a struggle. They have had to take sometimes painful steps to pay for care. They have borrowed money from a loved one, taken money out of a retirement account, or even taken a second mortgage on a home to pay medical bills. It is estimated that more than half of personal bankruptcies in the United States are a result of medical costs.

If you have difficulty paying bills, talk to someone. Many hospitals will work with you to arrange a payment plan that allows you to pay over time. Or they may be aware of programs in the community that can help.

"Contact your hospital or your doctors if you've got a lot of medical bills stacked up and work out a payment plan."
—Christy, head and neck cancer survivor

Even though the cost of care can be a challenge, help is out there. The resources at the end of this book (page 251) might be able to help with co-pays, out-of-pocket expenses, and other unanticipated costs. Don't ignore the problem. That can lead to higher bills and more anxiety. Get ahead of it and lean on those around you to help.

RESOURCES TO FOCUS ON FINANCES

The resources listed here offer general information about managing the cost of care. Refer to the back of this book for a list of resources for financial support. These organizations are here to help you. This is why they exist. Don't feel embarrassed or hesitate to call. Remember, most people with cancer are dealing with the same struggles—you are not alone.

Cancer Support Community's *Frankly Speaking About Cancer: Coping with the Cost of Care*—www.cancersupportcommunity.org/managing-cost-cancer-treatment

Cancer Support Community's "Managing the Cost of Cancer Treatment"—www.cancersupportcommunity.org/managing-cost-cancer-treatment

Triage Cancer—triagecancer.org

CHAPTER 23

Sex and Intimacy

When you are coping with cancer, sex might be the last thing on your mind. You may not feel well. Any energy you have is directed toward your own care and recovery. Yet, for many of us, sex is a vital part of who we are and how we express ourselves. The need for sex or intimacy can remain very present throughout the cancer experience. The absence of sex or intimacy can feel like a loss, which you grieve. Even if you do not feel this way, changes to a sex life can cause conflict between partners. If sexual side effects become a problem or add to your stress level, it is important to address them.

SEX

Issues with sex can be physical or psychological, or both. Some cancer treatments can reduce your sex drive or interfere with sexual function. Cancer can also cause physical changes that affect body image and lessen your interest in sex. Fatigue and depression can affect sex and intimacy as well. Depression can lessen your desire for sex, but some of the drugs used to treat it can decrease your libido. If you experience sexual side effects, the first step is to talk about it.

Start by talking with your doctor—perhaps your oncologist or primary care doctor. Men may consult a urologist, or women a gynecologist. A doctor can help you figure out the cause and possibly provide treatment to help. There are medicines to address sexual symptoms. A doctor can prescribe drugs for erectile dysfunction or hormones for vaginal lubrication. They also may recommend over-the-counter products like a lubricant from the drugstore.

If there is no physical cause, your doctor may recommend counseling or medications to help with depression. As mentioned, some drugs to treat depression can reduce desire for sex. If this is a concern, talk to your doctor about your reactions to antidepressants. Explore whether there are alternatives to combat depression, like therapy or natural remedies, that don't affect your sex drive.

Here are a few tips to keep in mind:[1]

- Talk with your health care team. The more you share, the more they can help you or the more equipped they will be to refer you to someone who can. They may be able to suggest or prescribe treatments for physical symptoms.

- Let your health care team know about any drugs or supplements you are trying. This includes prescription and over-the-counter medicines, and vitamins, herbs, and other supplements. Some may interfere with cancer treatment or have other risks.

- If you have a partner, talk with them about how you feel. Work together to determine how to deal with times when you may not be "in the mood." It is important to communicate with each other. These conversations can also help you become closer. If it's hard to talk about sexual issues, you may find couples therapy to be helpful.

- Remember that there are many ways to have sex and feel sexual. If you are struggling, find other ways to be intimate. Use your imagination and be creative!

---

1. Adapted from Cancer Support Community, *Frankly Speaking About Cancer: Metastatic Breast Cancer,* February 2019, www.cancersupportcommunity.org/mbc.

- You can feel intimacy in many different ways. Gentle touching, holding hands, kissing, and hugging can help you feel closer and more connected to another person.
- Other people with cancer may have tips to share. If you feel uncomfortable bringing up sex in a support group, ask the leader privately to raise the topic. You probably are not the only person with questions or concerns.
- If sex is important to you, and it's not getting better, you may want to seek help from a sex therapist or sexual health specialist.

INTIMACY

A cancer diagnosis can turn a household upside down. Roles shift, demands are heightened, and caregivers take on extra tasks and responsibilities. These disruptions, combined with the emotional toll of cancer, can affect your relationship with a spouse or partner. You and your partner may feel disconnected, even distant. It is critical to address these feelings up front before they fester. Resentment can build up and lead to even more conflict or distance.

If you are not sure how to express yourself, especially as it relates to sex or intimacy, you may want to consider couples counseling or a sex therapist. A counselor can bridge the communication gap. They can help you find the words and the courage to use the words needed to let your partner know how you are feeling. They may also be able to offer practical tips and exercises to try. Be open with your partner about your feelings and desires. Focus on listening to each other. Communication is key.

Some people find that, although they are not as interested in sex while they are in active treatment, their sexual desire returns after treatment ends and they recover more fully. Others feel self-conscious after cancer treatment due to a scar, hair loss, or other physical effects of cancer and its treatment. These feelings can affect intimacy.

Regardless of your situation, share your feelings with your partner and explore solutions together. We can't expect those we love to read our minds or anticipate our needs and desires. There will be ups and downs as time passes. Expressing your feelings and desires to your loved one, even when there are physical limitations to sex and intimacy, will help strengthen the bond between you and deepen your emotional connection to each other. Keep in mind that there are many ways to show love and affection. Consider other ways to give each other pleasure. Show tenderness through hugs, touching, and acts of kindness.

Some couples find it helpful to set time aside to be together. You may plan a date night, even if it means ordering in and watching a movie. Accept offers from friends or family to watch the kids for a few hours, or even overnight. It may be a fun distraction for the kids and give you time to be intimate or even just talk without distractions or fears of your conversations being overheard.

Know that you are not alone if you are struggling with intimacy related to cancer and cancer treatment. Take time to address these concerns with your partner and turn to others, whether they be professionals or peers, for help. Set aside time to talk to your partner and commit to open communication. It will be time well spent and can even be a part of your healing and wellness during and beyond cancer.

Sexuality Remains Neglected in Oncology Care

LESLIE R. SCHOVER, PhD

Dr. Schover is a clinical psychologist who has spent much of her career on research and clinical program development to help cancer patients and partners with problems of sexual function, intimacy, and fertility.

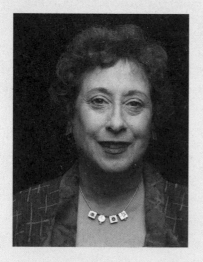

It may surprise you that problems with enjoying sex and functioning sexually are some of the most common unmet needs in repeated surveys of cancer survivors. In a recent study of more than ten thousand recently treated cancer patients in Canada, 43 percent reported having problems with sexual intimacy. Only 30 percent of people in this group had sought help. In fact, 70 percent still reported sexual intimacy to be unsatisfactory. Patients reported very similar findings regarding decreased sexual activity since their cancer diagnosis and treatment.

Sexual problems after cancer are often dismissed as "just emotional" because of a "damaged body image." The reality is that problems are caused by a damaged body. Some people lose a breast along with the pleasure of erotic sensation, or have to deal with an ostomy or incontinence during sex. Others do not have visible scars but lose desire for sex, have erection problems, or have pain during sex because cancer treatment affects the body systems needed for a healthy sexual response, including lowered hormone levels, damage to crucial nerves, and reduced blood flow to the sexual organs.

Even though the damage is physical, regaining a pleasurable sex life or getting through the stress of infertility treatment requires good emotional coping skills. For those in a committed relationship, the quality of intimacy, caring, and communication is also vital. That's why recent practice guidelines on sex and cancer from the American Society of Clinical Oncology call for multidisciplinary evaluation and treatment of problems.

Sadly, only about half of cancer patients recall any discussion of sexuality with a member of their oncology team. If sex is mentioned, it is typically the patient who raises the topic. The most common communication is a mention of possible sexual problems as part of the lengthy informed consent before treatment. When women with breast cancer, for example, asked about sexual problems, a "thorough" talk lasted about two minutes. It is probably not fair to expect oncologists or oncology nurses to keep sex on their radar screens. Appointment times are brief and crowded with many topics crucial to discuss. Other barriers to care for sexual problems in oncology settings include a lack of training for oncology professionals in the types and frequency of sexual problems, resulting in failure to recognize the prevalence and importance of sexual dysfunction. Only a few are comfortable discussing sex and cancer. Even fewer are familiar with options for medical and psychosocial care for sexual problems.

Specialists like psychologists, gynecologists, urologists, and pelvic rehabilitation–certified physical therapists often have limited knowledge and experience with post-cancer sexual problems. Experts tend to cluster in major cancer centers or at least large cities, making it difficult for many patients to find help. The surge in using telehealth visits may actually make it easier to find help from a trained professional. Insurance coverage may sometimes be limited, especially for mental health services like sexual counseling.

If you are experiencing a sexual problem related to your cancer treatment, you will probably have to be assertive to find good care. Bring up the problem with your oncology team and ask for referrals and resources. Trusted online cancer organizations may also have information on causes of problems and treatment options, and even lists of expert clinicians. Sexual health is a basic human right, even when a chronic health problem interferes.

RESOURCES FOR SEXUALITY AND INTIMACY

American Cancer Society's "Fertility and Sexual Side Effects in People with Cancer"—Covers topics related to sexuality, fertility, men, women, and the impact of different treatments. www.cancer.org/treatment/treatments-and-side-effects/physical-side-effects/fertility-and-sexual-side-effects.html

Cancer Support Community's *Frankly Speaking About Cancer: Your Relationship with Your Spouse or Partner*—www.cancersupportcommunity.org/intimacy-sex-and-fertility-issues

Cancer Support Community's "Intimacy, Sex and Fertility Issues"—www.cancersupport community.org/intimacy-sex-and-fertility-issues

Cancer Support Community's "Quality of Life for Cancer Patients"—Includes ten tips to help you regain your desire for sex after cancer. www.cancersupportcommunity.org/quality-life-cancer-patients

CHAPTER 24

Managing Work and Cancer

Work is a big part of life for many of us. You may feel a strong commitment to what you do, or you may see it mostly as a way to support yourself. Your job may be your passion or a daily grind. Either way, if you are employed when you learn you have cancer, you will have questions about your job. You may wonder if you can continue working through treatment. You may worry about money, sick time, or your rights as an employee.

The decision to keep working is a very personal one. It can have wide-ranging implications for you and your family. Some people continue working through treatment because it gives them a sense of normalcy and purpose. Others find continuing to work too stressful or perhaps physically impossible.

"My radiation treatment every morning was at seven fifteen or seven thirty. I would drive myself down there, put my face mask on, do the radiation, and then I would drive to work. I was a little late. The bank was most supportive. It's not a big national bank and everybody knew what I was going through. They said, 'You do what you have to do and when it's time for you to go home, you go home.' Well, I did. I kept working right up until the beginning of the six weeks and that's when I said, 'I can't take any more, guys.'"
—Bill, head and neck cancer survivor

If you are unable to work, the United States has some protections and safety nets in place to help you. Before we get to those, ask yourself these questions:

Things to Consider When Deciding Whether to Work Through Treatment[1]

- Do I enjoy my work and/or find it a welcome distraction?
- Have my career priorities changed?
- What does my health care team recommend?
- Can I complete my work functions while in treatment?
- What are the common side effects of my cancer treatment, and how might coping with them affect my work?
- How would taking time away from work affect my income?
- How much sick leave do I have?
- If I take time off from work, will the Family and Medical Leave Act apply?
- Do I live in a state with a state-sponsored short-term disability program?
- Do I have a disability insurance benefit through my employer? If so, how much will it pay?
- Do I have private disability insurance? If so, how much will it pay?

---

1. Adapted from Cancer Support Community, *Frankly Speaking About Cancer: Coping with the Cost of Care*, March 2020, www.cancersupportcommunity.org/managing-cost-cancer-treatment.

- Will I qualify for long-term Social Security Disability Insurance (SSDI)? If so, do I have savings to carry me through the five- to six-month waiting period?
- If I decide to stop working temporarily or permanently, how will this affect me and others?
- If I decide to stop working, what will I need to do to keep my health insurance?

One of the first decisions you may face is whether or when to tell your supervisor or coworkers about your cancer diagnosis. This is your choice, but some people find that telling people at work makes life easier. You can work together to adapt your workload, especially during active treatment. Leaning on others can help you feel supported and less stressed.

If you decide to work through treatment, you may need some flexibility. Your employer is required, under the **Americans with Disabilities Act (ADA)**, to provide what is referred to as "reasonable accommodation." This means your employer must make reasonable changes so you can do your job. For example, your supervisor might modify your schedule to accommodate medical treatments or allow you to work from home sometimes. It may mean making changes to your work space so you are more comfortable. The ADA is intended to protect people with disabilities, including cancer, from discrimination in the workplace. Take time to learn about it and understand how it protects you or your loved one.

---

*"I cried when I realized I had to leave my job of twenty years.
If I couldn't do the job I like, what would I do now? I've learned how to
grieve the loss of multiple events as a result of this disease."*
—Felicia, metastatic breast cancer survivor

If you find you are unable to work for a limited period of time, or even longer, look into your disability benefits. Explore whether your employer offers short- or long-term disability. Or perhaps you purchased disability insurance on your own. Disability insurance allows you to take time off from work for health reasons and receive a portion of your pay. The time allowed and percentage of pay you receive varies by policy.

If you have cancer or are caring for a loved one with cancer, you can also request time off through the **Family and Medical Leave Act (FMLA)**. This federal law allows an ill person, or the family member of an ill person, to take up to twelve weeks of leave without pay. The time can be taken all at once or in increments. While your employer is not required to pay you during this time, they are required to maintain your health benefits and preserve your job, or a job that is similar in pay and responsibilities.

You may find that you are unable to work at all and need to leave your job. If this happens, you may worry about losing your health insurance. In most cases, you can keep your health insurance for some time through the **Consolidated Omnibus Budget Reconciliation Act (COBRA)**. COBRA allows you to buy insurance through work after you leave your job for a certain period of time (often up to eighteen months). You will be responsible for 100 percent of the cost of the insurance. The monthly fee will be high, but COBRA allows you to maintain the coverage you know while you explore other options.

So, what are the other options? In 2010, Congress enacted the **Patient Protection and Affordable Care Act**, sometimes referred to as the ACA or Obamacare. The goal of the ACA is to make affordable health care available to the average American, based on income. The law created state-based exchanges or marketplaces where you can shop for health insurance. You can compare the plans offered in your state and their benefits. In this way, the ACA provides an open market for health insurance. If you leave work and are considering your options, look at the costs and benefits closely. The monthly premiums of an ACA plan are likely to be much lower than what you would pay through COBRA, but the benefits may be less, too. It is very important to research these plans carefully. Pay special attention to the details of the coverage. Ask yourself:

- Do my current doctors accept this insurance?
- Are my doctors in-network or out-of-network? This may affect your out-of-pocket costs.
- Will my medications be covered under the new plan?
- Will my routine scans and tests be covered under the new plan?
- How much will my deductibles be under the new plan?
- What are the co-payments for doctor visits, medications, tests, and scans?

Pay attention to all the costs. You may get excited about the prospect of low monthly premiums, but look at the whole picture. Out-of-pocket costs can be significant with some plans, especially for a serious diagnosis like cancer.

Another option is to apply for **Social Security Disability Insurance (SSDI)**. SSDI is a benefit provided by the federal government. It is designed for people who are not yet retirement age, have worked and paid into the Social Security system for years, and are now unable to work. To qualify for SSDI, you must be completely unable to work. You will need paperwork from your doctor to confirm that. The application process for SSDI is complex. It can take many months. If you apply, take your time completing the application. Fill in each field and answer each question carefully. Make sure that you include all the required documentation. Often, the application is returned because it is incomplete or missing attachments. If you can, try to find a social worker or lawyer to help you apply. If you are interested, get started right away. Try not to get frustrated, and understand that it will be a lengthy process.

In addition to SSDI, there is another federal program called **Supplemental Security Income (SSI)**. This program is for people who are older, blind or disabled, and have little to no income. It provides support for basics like food and housing. You can ask for assistance with this application, and the SSDI application, at your local Social Security office.

Understanding these laws and your work benefits may sound overwhelming. It's not you. They are complicated. Check to see if your employer has a human resources professional or benefits expert to help sort through your options. A hospital social worker may be able to help, too.

This is a good opportunity to call on your team for support. See if a close friend or family member might be able to help you learn about options and fill out forms.

Even though decisions related to work may feel daunting, it's a good idea to focus on this issue right away. Take time to make a decision that is right for you and your family. We list some excellent resources at the end of this chapter and the end of the book. They can help you learn more about your rights and the various laws in place to protect you. They also offer tips to manage employment and cancer. Also look for resources from your state, county, town, or city. They may offer support above and beyond the federal laws. Taking care of employment issues early on will leave you more time to focus on taking care of yourself later.

RESOURCES FOR MANAGING WORK AND CANCER

Cancer and Careers—Information for people with cancer in the workforce. www.cancer andcareers.org/en

Cancer Support Community's "Employment and Cancer"—Resources on work and cancer, including a webinar on managing work and cancer. www.cancersupport community.org/employment-and-cancer

Cancer Support Community's "Managing the Cost of Cancer Treatment"—Resource for insurance, employment, and managing the cost of care. www.cancersupport community.org/managing-cost-cancer-treatment

HealthCare.gov—Learn how to access health insurance in your state. www.healthcare .gov

Social Security Administration—Apply for benefits. www.ssa.gov

Triage Cancer's "Work and Employment"—Videos, webinars, and more related to work and cancer. triagecancer.org/cancer-employment-work-rights

CHAPTER 25

What If Treatment Doesn't End?

For many cancer patients, treatment has a beginning, a middle, and an end. You may be in treatment for weeks or months, but there is a light at the end of the tunnel. For others, treatment continues for many months or even years. And, for some, treatment becomes a permanent part of life.

Imagining yourself in treatment for such a long period of time can bring mixed emotions and a new set of practical challenges. Some people say they are happy and relieved that there continue to be treatment options for them. This was not the case even a generation ago. For some, treatment manages to keep the cancer under control for long periods of time, adding truth to the idea of cancer as a chronic disease. While that is a step in the right direction, months or years of cancer treatment can take an emotional and financial toll. It affects the way people think about their lives and interact with others.

In this chapter, we focus on the challenge of coping with cancer that doesn't go away. If you find yourself here, it may be because your cancer is metastatic or advanced. Or you may have an early-stage or slow-growing cancer that does not need treatment right now but probably will at some point. This is often true of smoldering multiple myeloma, chronic lymphocytic leukemia (CLL), and other blood cancers.

METASTATIC CANCER

If you are diagnosed with metastatic cancer, or cancer that has spread to other parts of the body, the news can be devastating. Yet, thanks to advances in treatment, people with metastatic disease live longer and more comfortably than ever before. Take breast cancer, for example. We have seen a steady increase in survival rates for people with metastatic or advanced breast cancer. Many live years beyond diagnosis.

Now that there are more treatments for patients with advanced cancer, people sometimes stay with one treatment for as long as it works. If it stops controlling the cancer, they move on to another treatment. Some may try several different treatments over time. They may try both standard treatments and clinical trials.

Regardless of your path, advanced cancer can evoke many emotions, such as fear, uncertainty, and anxiety. If you are in this situation, it is important to slow down and focus on one step at a time. Consider your priorities. Think about what really matters to you. You may find more joy in small things and put more energy into the people and activities you love. You may think about the legacy you want to leave behind for family or others—and invest in that legacy. You may find yourself making photo albums, telling your life story in writing or on video, or thinking about your ethical will or the life lessons you want to convey. This also may be a time to connect with others and nurture the relationships that mean the most to you.

SLOW-GROWING CANCER

The treatment for chronic cancers, like multiple myeloma or CLL, varies widely depending on the type and stage of disease. Some patients proceed right away to targeted therapy or chemotherapy. For others, doctors may recommend a stem cell transplant. Or they might suggest "watch and wait," which we mentioned in chapter four. This approach involves regular monitoring. You do not start any type of treatment right away.

Watch and wait, also referred to as active surveillance or watchful waiting, can be stressful or upsetting. It can be hard to know that you have cancer but are not treating it. The decision to watch and wait is used most often with blood cancers and early-stage prostate, breast, and thyroid cancers. Here are some tips for coping with watch and wait:

Tips for Coping with Watchful Waiting[1]

- Ask your health care team questions until you understand why watchful waiting is a good choice for you. Remember that you, too, are a key member of your team, so speak up if you have questions or concerns.

- Ask your health care team about all the treatment options that are available to you, including clinical trials. It is important that you understand them so you and your health care team can make decisions together about the best choices for you.

- Learn and recognize any signs or symptoms you should tell your health care team about right away.

- Find out if there are any biomarkers or lab tests that will be used to monitor your cancer.

- Accept that you do not have control over some aspects of your cancer.

- Keep written notes about signs or symptoms you notice and any other questions you have. Take notes during your conversations with your health care team. You may find it useful to bring someone with you to your medical appointments.

- Know that you will be more anxious when it gets closer to your doctor's appointments. Be gentle with yourself when you are feeling stressed.

- Yoga, breathing, relaxation exercises, and doing activities you enjoy can help you relax.

- Focus on what gives you pleasure now, instead of worrying about the future. Make time for what you really want. Pamper yourself in small ways—take a warm bath, read a good book, or buy yourself a small gift.

- Know that it's normal to have fears, but practice letting them go. Try to picture them floating away, being washed away, being vaporized, or leaving as you breathe out.

---

1. Adapted from Cancer Support Community, *Frankly Speaking About Cancer: Coping with Chronic Lymphocytic Leukemia (CLL)*, December 2018, www.cancersupportcommunity.org/cll.

"I was waiting for the other shoe to drop. When I relapsed, I was devastated but also relieved. The shoe had dropped and now we could deal with it."
—Jen, acute myeloid leukemia survivor

Managing a chronic cancer can take an emotional toll on patients and families. Sometimes, it is hard to adapt to the idea of cancer never going away. Endless treatments, scans, and medical appointments become regular reminders of cancer. It might sound clichéd, but the old saying "live in the moment" may apply here more than ever. Try not to let cancer consume your life or thoughts. Continue to do the things you love and explore new interests. Make plans for future events, activities, or trips. Find ways to take back some control of your life. If this sounds impossible, consider seeking support or trying the mind-body approaches discussed in chapter twenty-one.

Some people tell us that having a chronic cancer affects the way they interact with others. For example, you may look well; perhaps you have not lost your hair and have no outward signs of illness. But you don't feel well. People may assume that you are better or that treatment has ended. This places the burden on you to share how you are feeling with those around you. This can be hard to do but is often worth the effort. You may gain support and strengthen relationships when you are honest about your limitations.

"A lot of people don't know much about metastatic breast cancer. They believe you can't really be sick if you don't look sick."
—Amanda, metastatic breast cancer survivor

A chronic cancer can also be a financial drain on you and your family. Years of medical care can mean years of co-pays, deductibles, and other out-of-pocket costs. Take time to review chapters nine and twenty-two about health insurance and finances, respectively. They provide helpful tips and strategies to help with long-term planning. If you have a financial adviser, you may want to speak to them as well.

Chronic cancer can prompt people to make lifestyle changes. You may want to focus on staying as strong and healthy as possible. This can be an opportunity to seek help quitting smoking, increasing exercise, or making healthier food choices. Be sure to pull out the insert in this book for recipes that are packed full of vitamins and other nutrients.

Lastly, whether you are dealing with metastatic disease or a chronic cancer, you may want to talk with others who are in the same or a similar situation. Consider finding a support group, asking your health care team to introduce you to other patients, or looking for ways to connect online through chat rooms and digital discussion boards. Others in your situation can empathize, offer tips, or just be good listeners. Even when you have a strong support network, talking to someone who knows what you are going through can be both reassuring and comforting.

"When I've had recurrences, I imagine the timeline of my life. Here's the first diagnosis and that was a big speed bump. I didn't think it would ever get better, and life would never be the same, but it was. Each time, I take myself back to the first time, the worst ever memory of how it felt. I thought it was never going to get better, and it did, it did get better with each time. I'm happy to be here and I'm happy to live with it and I adjust as I need to, to adapt to the way my life is today and I'm thankful for the way it is."

—Christy, head and neck cancer survivor

RESOURCES

Cancer Support Community's "Active Surveillance"—www.cancersupportcommunity
.org/active-surveillance

Leukemia and Lymphoma Society's "Watch and Wait"—www.lls.org/treatment/types-of
-treatment/watch-and-wait

Metastatic Breast Cancer Network (MBCN)—A patient-led advocacy organization that
educates, advocates, and empowers. 888-500-0370 or www.mbcn.org

AFTER TREATMENT IS DONE

CHAPTER 26

Tools for Survivorship and Beyond

You've had your last infusion or your last round of radiation. Treatment is over. You've looked forward to this day for weeks or months. You may have counted down on a calendar. You imagined this as the time when life would return to normal—as it was before. As this day brings relief, it may bring other feelings as well. The transition from cancer patient to cancer survivor can be stressful. This time can present a whole new spectrum of emotions and fears. It can be difficult to lose frequent contact with your medical team. While visits to the doctor for checkups, scans, and chemo were challenging, they also may have brought comfort and provided a safety net. They were a source of support.

People who have been through this experience describe many of the same worries. They include:

- Will my cancer come back?
- How do I manage the changes to my body?

- Will the side effects I am still experiencing go away, or will they linger for a long period of time?
- How do I recover from the financial impact cancer has had on me and my family?
- How do I use my cancer experience to make meaningful changes in my life?
- Do I want to go back to work?
- Which doctors should I now see and how often?

"I felt lost after treatment was over. The psychological blinders most people wear to avoid seeing how fragile and fleeting life can be were off and I was left with the question of what to do with the new life I was given to live."
—Andy, acute myeloid leukemia survivor

WHO IS A CANCER SURVIVOR?[1]

The National Cancer Institute defines a cancer survivor as "anyone who has been diagnosed with cancer from the time of diagnosis until the end of their life." The Centers for Disease Control and Prevention extend the definition to include family members, friends, and caregivers who are affected by a cancer diagnosis.

---

1. "Cancer Transitions," Cancer Support Community, accessed October 21, 2020, www.cancersupportcommunity.org/cancer-transitions.

In years past, the concerns of people who completed treatment were often ignored or overlooked. After treatment ended, patients no longer saw an oncologist on a regular basis. Their primary care doctor was not aware of the details of their cancer treatment. This doctor was not familiar with the potential long-term side effects and increased risks.

Then, in 2006, the Institute of Medicine (IOM) issued a report called *From Cancer Patient to Cancer Survivor: Lost in Transition.* The report outlines the needs of cancer survivors and offers ten recommendations on caring for them.

The report states: "The transition from active treatment to post-treatment care is critical to long-term health. If care is not planned and coordinated, cancer survivors are left without knowledge of their heightened risks and a follow-up plan of action. However, such a plan is essential so that routine follow-up visits become opportunities to promote a healthy lifestyle, check for cancer recurrence, and manage lasting effects of the cancer experience."[2] The authors of the report describe its aims as follows:

1. Raise awareness of the medical, functional, and psychosocial consequences of cancer and its treatment.
2. Define quality health care for cancer survivors and identify strategies to achieve it.
3. Improve the quality of life of cancer survivors through policies to ensure their access to psychosocial services, fair employment practices, and health insurance.[3]

Their point was clear. People with cancer need support and resources to transition from patient to survivor. This report marked a turning point for people who had cancer. Survivorship was finally understood as a distinct phase of cancer care. The unique needs of survivors were outlined in writing and recognized by doctors and health care organizations.

But what does this mean for you as you make the transition from patient to survivor? To get started, here are some actions you can take as you plan for this next phase of life:

---

2. Institute of Medicine and National Resource Council, *From Cancer Patient to Cancer Survivor: Lost in Transition,* The National Academies Press (2006), 1, https://doi.org/10.17226/11468.

3. Institute of Medicine and National Resource Council, *From Cancer Patient to Cancer Survivor,* 2.

Ten Actions for Survivors[4]

1. *Stay in the moment.* Try to focus on resolving only today's problems—take a deep breath and take one step at a time.

2. *Help others understand what you need.* Let friends and family know what would help you. Many people want to help but are unsure of what you want. Make specific suggestions, such as, "Let's go to a movie," or "I need you to hold me and just listen when I talk," or "I could really use some help with the kids tomorrow when I have my appointment with the doctor."

3. *Acknowledge your feelings.* The cancer experience triggers many strong emotions. The first step is to take time to just listen to your body and to the things you are saying to yourself in your mind. Once you are more aware of your feelings, you can find constructive ways to express them through talking, writing, physical activity, or creative pursuits. Some people are more private than others, but opening up to someone you trust can help.

4. *Do what you enjoy.* If you are still able to participate in activities you enjoyed before the diagnosis, keep doing them. Ask friends to join you or give yourself permission to be alone when you need to be.

5. *Seek relaxation.* "Relaxation" refers to a calm, controlled physical state that will enhance your well-being. The more you practice relaxation, the easier it becomes. Each of us can find ways to take relaxing breaks in our daily routine. Listen to some music that moves your spirit. Do a few stretches. Take time to enjoy some scenery. Consider joining a relaxation or meditation program in your community. Even watching your favorite TV show can put you in a relaxed state.

6. *Retain as much control of your life as is reasonable.* If you feel that you have lost control to health professionals, loved ones, or even the disease itself, list things you feel you have lost control of—then decide what you can realistically take back. Even the simplest things can help enhance your sense of control.

---

4. "Cancer Transitions," Cancer Support Community.

7. *Maintain a partnership with your doctor.* Aim for ongoing communication and never stop asking questions through the period of follow-up care and into the future.

8. *Be an empowered survivor.* Be an active participant in the care of your mind and body. If you feel better about your choices, you will improve the quality of your life.

9. *Spend time with other cancer survivors.* People with cancer often find a sense of comfort in communicating with others who share their experiences in person, online, or by phone. Cancer support organizations, such as the Cancer Support Community, can help you connect with other cancer survivors.

10. *Hope for many things.* Hope is desirable and reasonable. There are millions of people in the world today for whom cancer is just a memory. Even if your cancer recovery is complicated, you can find small goals and pleasures in your life. Get tickets to a concert. Look forward to a Bible study class. Make a special effort to be present for a family event, like a birthday or anniversary of someone you love. Look forward to your hair growing back. People who find something that gives them hope are often better equipped to handle whatever challenges lie ahead. Talk about what gives you hope and what you hope for, now and in the future.

The Cancer Support Community has a program called Cancer Transitions that helps patients make the transition from cancer patient to cancer survivor in a meaningful and structured way. The program focuses on four key areas: (1) psychosocial health, (2) eating well, (3) staying active, and (4) medical management. A little later in this chapter, we will review the first three items in greater depth. We will address the fourth item, medical management, more thoroughly in chapter twenty-seven.

Before we get into specifics, let's pause for a moment. As you think about a personalized plan for this next stage of life, it is easy to get overwhelmed. It's tempting to try to do too many things at once. By pacing yourself, you can make realistic plans that will work for you. Use the SMART tips in this chapter to help.

CREATING A HEALTHY LIFESTYLE PLAN[5]

Being a cancer survivor can be overwhelming. For the first time in a long time, you are solely in charge of your health in a way that is not possible during treatment. It is time for you to take back control. A healthy lifestyle, which includes nutritious foods and physical activity, is a great way to begin. Work with your health care team to make a plan that is right for you. Start with small changes. Set a goal to keep yourself on track. A good rule of thumb to remember is to make your goals SMART.

- **S**—Set **specific** goals because general goals are much harder to achieve. For example, instead of "I will go to the gym," try "I will go to the gym two days during the week and one day on the weekend."

- **M**—Set **measurable** goals. Goals are easier to work on when they are concrete. Instead of saying "I will eat more fruits and vegetables," try "I will eat five different fruits and vegetables each day."

- **A**—Set **attainable** goals that make sense for you and your current lifestyle. Don't be afraid to be bold and try something new. For example, "try one new recipe each week" might be an attainable goal for you if you have the energy and enjoy cooking. If you don't like to cook, try to make a new smoothie instead. Smoothies can be made easily in a blender.

- **R**—Set **realistic** goals that are doable for you at this stage in your cancer journey. If you've just completed treatment and are still dealing with some ongoing side effects like fatigue, cooking a healthy dinner from scratch every night might not be a realistic goal. Instead, make one recipe, like marinated grilled chicken breasts, that can be repurposed in meals throughout the week.

----

5. Adapted from "Cancer Transitions," Cancer Support Community.

> • **T**—Set **timely** goals. A time frame can help you stay on track. For example, if you often skip meals, it might be helpful to set certain times of the day to eat breakfast, lunch, and dinner. Regular meals will help you avoid excess hunger and overeating.

Some people see ending cancer treatment as a chance to make sweeping lifestyle changes. They intend to turn over a new leaf. As you consider your next steps, remember the SMART tips.

Taking on too much all at once can lead to failure and disappointment. It might derail you from your plan. Set smaller goals that grow over time. Consider asking a family member or friend to join you in your effort. The buddy system works and can help you stay motivated and on track.

Here are some more factors to consider as you transition to survivorship:

Emotional health and well-being: Completing cancer treatment can bring mixed emotions ranging from fear and uncertainty to relief and gratitude. Just because you are done with treatment doesn't necessarily mean you are done with cancer. It is important to acknowledge your emotions and find ways and places to process them. You may want to find a survivorship group in your community or online, or practice some of the mind-body and wellness techniques we reviewed in chapter twenty-one. Fear that the cancer will return is one of the greatest concerns survivors raise. For some, it can be debilitating. We will discuss that more in chapter twenty-eight and suggest ways to manage the fear.

Exercise: Many people see survivorship as a chance to get back to an exercise routine they loved, create a modified routine that takes into consideration the changes in their bodies, or start a brand-new routine that works for them. Exercise can help with both physical *and* mental health and can help you take back some control of your life. Exercise can also help you rebuild muscle tone and achieve a healthy weight. Be sure to consult with your doctor if you are embarking on a new routine and be kind to yourself. Recognize your limitations and set small goals that you can achieve and celebrate.

Nutrition: A heathy diet is another way to take back some control after treatment and make lifestyle changes that you deem important. A well-balanced diet can help with recovery: it can boost your immune system and help you build your strength back up. A diet rich in lean proteins, whole grains, and healthy fruits and vegetables can fuel your survivorship and lead to a better quality of life. Learning about nutrition and cooking can be a great family activity that is both fun and educational. Be sure to check out the healthy recipes in the pullout of this book.

Use your post-treatment phase as a chance to regain some control, find new meaning in your life, and set goals that align with your values and aspirations. Also, take this opportunity to connect with those you care about in new ways and set goals for a better future. You have the power and the strength to write your next chapter. Make it count!

RESOURCES FOR SURVIVORSHIP

Cancer Support Community's "Cancer Survivorship"—Support and resources for cancer survivors. www.cancersupportcommunity.org/cancer-survivorship

Cancer Support Community's "Cancer Transitions"—A comprehensive program designed to give you the energy and ability to cope with life after treatment. The program covers psychosocial health, eating well, staying active, and medical management. www.cancersupportcommunity.org/cancer-transitions

Livestrong's *The Road to Survivorship: Living After Cancer Treatment*—An overview from Livestrong of the physical, emotional, and practical issues faced by people who have experienced cancer treatment. Available in four languages and eleven cultural adaptations and in adolescent and LGBT versions. www.livestrong.org/what-we-do /living-after-cancer-treatment-brochure

National Cancer Institute's "Facing Forward: Life After Cancer Treatment"—www.cancer .gov/publications/patient-education/facing-forward

National Coalition for Cancer Survivorship's Cancer Survival Toolbox—Read and listen to articles on topics related to living with and beyond cancer. 877-NCCS-YES (877-622-7937) or www.canceradvocacy.org/resources/cancer-survival-toolbox

Colorful Fruits and Vegetables Provide Phytonutrients

Color		Example of Foods	Helpful Phytonutrients	Recipes
RED		Cherries and citrus fruit peel	Terpenes (such as perillyl alcohol, limonene, carnosol) help strengthen the immune system and fight off viruses.	**Fruit and Nut Bars** (cherries)
		Tomatoes and watermelon	Carotenoids (such as beta-carotene, lycopene, lutein, zeaxanthin) help boost your immune system.	**Quinoa Tabbouleh** (tomato)
BLUE AND PURPLE		Grapes and berries	Polyphenols (such as ellagic acid and resveratrol) can help prevent inflammation.	**Pear and Blueberry Crumble** (berries) **Mixed Berry and Yogurt Crepes** (berries)
GREEN		Cruciferous vegetables (such as broccoli, cabbage, collard greens, kale, and Brussels sprouts)	Isothiocyanates, indoles, and glucosinolates (sulforaphane) help reduce heart risk and protect against certain cancers.	**Lemon Parmesan Chicken with Broccoli Rice** (broccoli) **Kiwi Green Smoothie** (kale)
ORANGE		Carrots, apricots, cantaloupe, mangos, and oranges	Carotenoids (such as beta-carotene, lycopene, lutein, zeaxanthin) may reduce heart risk and boost your immune system.	**Shrimp Bento Bowl** (carrots) **Whitefish Tacos with Strawberry Mango Salsa** (mangos)
WHITE		Onions, soybeans, and soy products (tofu, soy milk, edamame, etc.)	Flavonoids (such as anthocyanins and quercetin) help prevent inflammation and reduce blood pressure.	**Swiss and Spinach Strata** (onion)
BLACK/BROWN		Cocoa and dates	Flavonoids (procyanidin) help reduce blood pressure.	**Chocolate Mint Smoothie** (cocoa) **Chocolate Hummus** (cocoa and dates) **Chocolate Hazelnut Spread** (chocolate/cocoa)

FRUIT AND NUT BARS

Prep time: 15 minutes   **Cooking time:** 15 minutes

1 cup chopped almonds
⅓ cup chopped cashews
¼ cup dried cherries
¼ cup dried apricots
½ cup unsweetened coconut flakes
2 tablespoons ground flaxseeds

2 tablespoons nut butter
¼ cup honey
1 tablespoon coconut oil

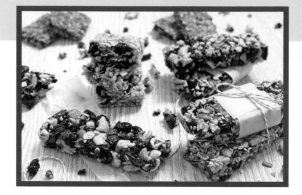

1 Preheat oven to 325°F. Line an 8 × 8 dish with parchment paper.

2 Combine nuts, dried fruit, coconut, and flax-seeds in a medium-sized bowl.

3 In a microwave-safe bowl, combine nut butter, honey, and coconut oil. Place in microwave to melt ingredients, 30 seconds to 1 minute. Add nut, fruit, and seed mixture and stir together.

4 Pour batter in prepared dish and spread out until smooth.

5 Bake in preheated oven for 15 minutes. Remove and let cool completely.

6 Cut into bars and store in refrigerator.

Tip: If you have leftovers, crumble a bar over oatmeal or yogurt.

QUINOA TABBOULEH

Prep time: 15 minutes   **Cooking time:** 15 minutes

1 cup quinoa, uncooked
1 cup diced tomatoes
1 cup diced cucumbers
½ cup diced red bell peppers
1 cup fresh parsley, chopped
½ cup fresh mint

2 lemons, juiced
2 tablespoons olive oil
½ cup feta cheese
   (optional)

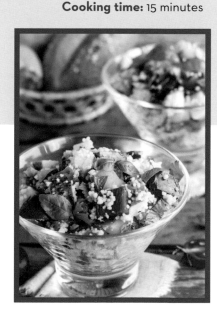

1 Rinse and cook quinoa according to package instructions.

2 While quinoa is on the stove, combine the tomatoes, cucumbers, peppers, and herbs in a large bowl.

3 Once quinoa is cooked and cooled, add to the vegetable and herb bowl.

4 Add lemon juice and olive oil.

5 Top with feta cheese if desired.

PEAR AND BLUEBERRY CRUMBLE

Prep time: 15 minutes

Cooking time: 25 minutes

4 pears, thinly sliced
2 cups blueberries
1 tablespoon pure maple syrup
2 teaspoons lemon juice
2 tablespoons whole wheat flour
2 tablespoons ground flaxseeds
½ cup old-fashioned oats

½ cup almonds, thinly chopped
¼ cup brown sugar
½ teaspoon ground cinnamon
¼ cup cold unsalted butter,
   cut into small cubes

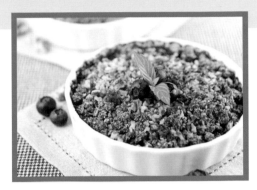

1 Preheat oven to 400°F.
2 Mix fruit, maple syrup, and lemon juice in a bowl.
3 Grease an 8 × 8 dish and add fruit mixture.
4 In a separate bowl, combine flour, flaxseeds, oats, almonds, brown sugar, and cinnamon.
5 Add butter to dry mixture and mix with your hands or wooden spoon until butter is combined with oat mixture.
6 Top fruit with oat mixture.
7 Bake, uncovered, for 20 to 25 minutes, until top is lightly browned.

Tip: Sprinkle leftover crumble on top of yogurt, oatmeal, or cottage cheese for a healthy and flavorful breakfast.

MIXED BERRY AND YOGURT CREPES

Prep time: 50 minutes (includes 30 minutes for batter to rest)

Cooking time: 25 minutes

3 eggs
1 cup milk
¼ cup water
½ cup all-purpose flour
½ cup whole wheat flour
¼ teaspoon salt

2 tablespoons canola oil
2 tablespoons pure maple syrup
1 cup vanilla yogurt
2 cups frozen mixed berries,
   thawed
1 teaspoon ground cinnamon

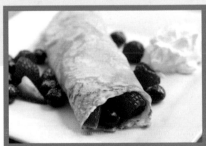

1 Whisk together eggs, milk, and water. Add both flours to wet ingredients and mix together gently.
2 Add salt, oil, and maple syrup to batter. Mix to combine.
3 Let batter rest for 30 minutes.
4 After rest time, lightly grease skillet and heat over low heat. Pour ¼ cup of batter into pan. Swirl it around to get batter to spread over the skillet.
5 Cook for 30 seconds to 1 minute then flip crepe over. To do this, loosen crepe with a spatula and quickly flip.
6 Cook on the other side for an additional 30 seconds.
7 Repeat with remaining batter.
8 Spoon a dollop of vanilla yogurt and fruit inside each crepe. Sprinkle lightly with cinnamon and roll crepe like a burrito to serve.

LEMON PARMESAN CHICKEN WITH BROCCOLI RICE

Prep time: 30 minutes (does not include chicken marinating time)   **Cooking time:** 15 minutes

2 tablespoons olive oil, divided
2 garlic cloves, minced, divided
2 ½ lemons, zested and juiced
1 teaspoon honey
1 ½ pounds boneless, skinless chicken breast
Salt and black pepper to taste

½ cup Parmesan cheese, divided
1 bunch broccoli

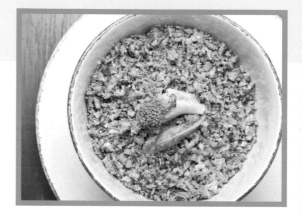

1   In a bowl or zip-top bag, combine 1 tablespoon olive oil, 1 minced garlic clove, lemon juice and zest, and honey.

2   Marinate chicken in mixture for 1 to 2 hours.

3   After marinating time, heat remaining olive oil in a pan over medium heat. Place chicken in heated pan and season with salt and pepper. Reserve marinade.

4   Cook chicken for 3 to 4 minutes on each side. Pour reserved marinade into pan and deglaze. Cook for 1 minute and add ¼ cup Parmesan.

5   While the chicken is cooking, make the broccoli rice. Roughly chop broccoli and add to a food processor. Process until broccoli is in small pieces, similar to rice.

6   In another pan, gently cook the remaining minced clove of garlic. Add riced broccoli and salt and pepper, and cook for 5 minutes. Add 2 tablespoons Parmesan and a squirt of remaining ½ lemon. Stir to combine.

7   Place broccoli rice in a bowl and top with cooked chicken and remaining Parmesan cheese.

KIWI GREEN SMOOTHIE

Prep time: 5 minutes   **Cooking time:** 0 minutes

2 kiwis
1 banana
½ cup plain Greek yogurt

1 tablespoon honey
1 cup fresh kale
1 cup 2% milk

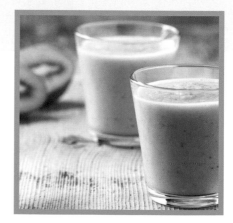

1   Place all ingredients in high-powered blender.

2   Blend until smooth.

Tip: Freeze leftover smoothie in a popsicle mold for a delicious summer treat!

SHRIMP BENTO BOWL

Prep time: 20 minutes   **Cooking time:** 0 minutes

¼ cup low sodium soy sauce (see tip)
1 tablespoon rice vinegar
1 inch fresh ginger, grated
1 tablespoon honey
2 cups cooked brown rice
1 cup diced cucumber

1 avocado, diced
1 carrot, cut into matchsticks
1 pound small cooked shrimp, peeled and tails removed
Sriracha sauce (optional)

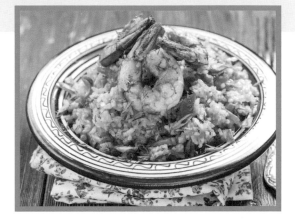

1. To make dressing, mix soy sauce, vinegar, ginger, and honey together in a small bowl.

2. To assemble your bento bowl, place brown rice in a bowl and top with vegetables and shrimp.

3. Toss with dressing and top with Sriracha sauce if desired.

Tip: You may reduce the soy sauce or replace with liquid aminos or homemade soy sauce as needed for less sodium content.

WHITE FISH TACOS WITH STRAWBERRY MANGO SALSA

Prep time: 10 minutes   **Cooking time:** 15 minutes

¼ cup orange juice
1 tablespoon honey
1 teaspoon ground cumin
1 teaspoon paprika
½ teaspoon salt
¼ teaspoon black pepper
1 pound cod or other white fish
½ cup strawberries, diced

1 mango, diced
¼ cup chopped cilantro
¼ cup chopped red cabbage
1 lime, juiced
½ jalapeno (optional)
1 tablespoon olive oil
8 corn tortillas

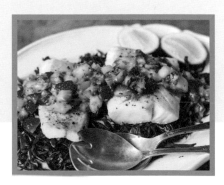

1. Combine orange juice, honey, cumin, paprika, and salt and pepper in a large container. Add fish to mixture and marinate for 10 minutes.

2. While the fish is marinating, make the fruit salsa. Combine strawberries, mango, cilantro, cabbage, lime juice, and jalapeno if desired. Store in the refrigerator until ready to use.

3. After the fish has marinated, heat olive oil in large skillet. Add fish to heated skillet and cook for 4 to 5 minutes on each side, brushing marinade onto the fish as it cooks.

4. Once fish is cooked, heat corn tortillas in microwave for 15 seconds, wrapped in a damp paper towel or clean dish towel.

5. When you are ready to eat, make your taco. Add fish to the corn tortilla and top with fruit salsa.

Tip: Use leftover fruit salsa to top chicken, vegetables, or black beans for a quick lunch or dinner.

SWISS AND SPINACH STRATA

Prep time: 20 minutes (does not include time resting overnight)   **Cooking time:** 45 minutes

1 tablespoon olive oil
1 onion, diced
1 garlic clove, minced
10 ounces frozen spinach, thawed and drained
8 slices whole wheat crusty bread, cubed
2 ½ cups milk
1 teaspoon salt

½ teaspoon black pepper
9 eggs
¾ cup grated Swiss cheese
¼ cup grated Parmesan cheese

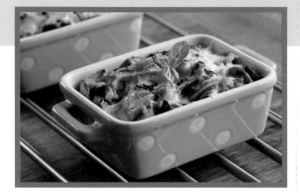

The day before serving:

1   Heat olive oil in a skillet over medium heat.

2   Add onion and cook for 5 minutes, until translucent. Add garlic and sauté for 1 minute. Add spinach and cook for 2 to 3 minutes. Set aside.

3   Grease a ceramic dish with nonstick spray. Add bread cubes and cooked spinach. Mix until combined.

4   In a separate bowl, combine milk, salt and pepper, eggs, and cheese. Pour egg mixture over bread and spinach.

5   Cover and place in the refrigerator overnight.

The next morning:

1   Preheat the oven to 375°F. Remove strata from refrigerator while oven is preheating.

2   Uncover and bake in oven for 45 to 50 minutes, until top is slightly browned.

CHOCOLATE MINT SMOOTHIE

Prep time: 5 minutes   **Cooking time:** 0 minutes

2 cups chocolate almond milk
1 tablespoon peanut butter
1 tablespoon unsweetened cocoa powder
5 to 8 mint leaves (depending on size
   and how minty you want the smoothie)
1 cup oats, uncooked

1 avocado
1 cup ice

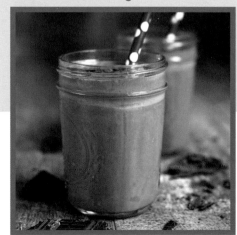

1   Place all ingredients in high-powered blender.

2   Blend until smooth.

Tip: If you have leftover smoothie, pour into popsicle mold for a refreshing and delicious treat!

CHOCOLATE HUMMUS

Prep time: 10 minutes

1 can chickpeas, drained
3 Medjool dates
¼ cup unsweetened cocoa powder
3 tablespoons honey
1 tablespoon pure maple syrup
⅓ cup smooth peanut butter

Cooking time: 0 minutes

½ teaspoon salt
¼ teaspoon vanilla extract
¼ to ½ cup water

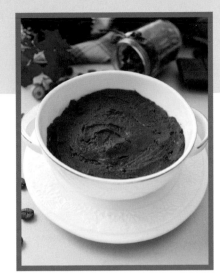

1 Combine all ingredients in a food processor or blender. Start with ¼ cup of water and increase based on desired consistency.

2 Serve with apples, strawberries, grapes, or cracker of your choice.

CHOCOLATE HAZELNUT SPREAD

Prep time: 5 minutes

2 cups raw hazelnuts
½ cup dark chocolate chips
½ teaspoon almond extract

Cooking time: 25 minutes

¼ to ½ teaspoon sea salt, depending on taste preference

1 Preheat oven to 350°F.

2 Spread raw hazelnuts on a baking sheet and roast in preheated oven for 12 minutes.

3 Remove roasted hazelnuts from oven and let slightly cool. Once slightly cooled, rub the hazelnuts in a clean dish towel to loosen the skins (some skin on the hazelnuts is okay).

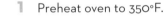

4 Blend hazelnuts in high-powered blender or food processor until they form a nut butter, about 8 minutes.

5 While blending hazelnuts, melt dark chocolate chips in microwave in 30-second increments, stirring after each increment.

6 Add melted chocolate, almond extract, and salt to the hazelnut butter. Process until smooth.

7 Serve with whole grain toast, fruit, or spooned on top of yogurt or ice cream.

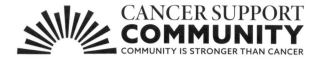

The Cancer Support Community (CSC) is a global nonprofit network that operates at 175 locations, including CSC and Gilda's Club centers, and in multiple hospitals and cancer clinics. Combined with a toll-free helpline, educational materials, and digital platforms, this network of professionally led services provides more than $50 million each year in free support and navigation to patients and families.

Formed in 2009 by the merger of The Wellness Community and Gilda's Club, CSC also conducts cutting-edge research on the emotional, psychological, and financial journey of cancer patients. In addition, CSC advocates at all levels of government for policies to help individuals whose lives have been disrupted by cancer. In January 2018, CSC welcomed Denver-based nonprofit MyLifeLine, a digital community that includes more than 40,000 patients, caregivers, and their supporters, enabling CSC to scale its digital services in innovative, groundbreaking ways. For more information, visit www.Cancer SupportCommunity.org. *So that no one faces cancer alone*®.

Visit CSC's online kitchen in our Virtual Home where you can explore more healthy recipes and cooking videos specifically created to support the nutritional needs of people impacted by cancer at https://www.cancersupportcommunity.org/virtual-programs.

The Cancer Support Helpline is here to make sure you find answers to your questions and concerns. Whether you are looking for nutrition advice, financial navigation, or need emotional support, call our Helpline at 1-888-793-9355.

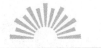

CHAPTER 27

Survivor Care Plan and Medical Follow-Up

W hen you have cancer, the rhythm of treatment—doctors, clinics, infusions, scans—is central to your days. Then it ends. We've talked about how this transition can affect your emotions. In this chapter, we address what it may mean for your health. Many survivors share that, after cancer treatment ends, they are unclear about what to do next, medically. They don't recall all the details of their cancer care, like the dates of surgeries or the names of the chemo drugs they were given. They aren't sure how often to return to the oncologist for follow-up care. Survivors are also sometimes uncertain of which doctor to see for what. Do you go back to the oncologist if you have lingering symptoms or side effects? What do you do if you have a cold? Or high blood pressure?

In chapter twenty-six, we discussed the Institute of Medicine (IOM) report *From Cancer Patient to Cancer Survivor: Lost in Transition*. One of the key recommendations of this report is that every patient, when completing treatment, should receive a survivor care plan. The IOM says:

> Recommendation Two: Patients completing primary treatment should be provided with a comprehensive care summary and follow-up plan that is clearly and effectively explained. This "Survivorship Care Plan" should be written by the principal provider(s) who coordinated oncology treatment. This service should be reimbursed by third-party payors of health care.[1]

But what should be included in the plan? Different hospitals and cancer centers use different survivor care plans. They are sometimes called treatment summaries or follow-up care plans. Even if your treatment center does not use a special template or form, you can ask for the information. This information will be a valuable record for you and your doctors. Make sure to share it with your primary care doctor and any specialists you see.

Here are some of the basics the plan may include:

- Details about your medical team and the location where you received care—for example, the name of the hospital or cancer center, and names and contact information for everyone involved in your care, including doctors, nurses, social workers, nutritionists, physical therapists, and so on
- The exact type and subtype of your cancer
- The stage or grade of disease
- Hormonal status
- Results and copies of all tests, scans, and so on
- Dates and details of surgeries
- Dates and details of radiation treatments
- Names and details of all medications you received and any you are still taking, including schedules, doses, frequency, and number of cycles
- Records and discharge reports of any emergency room visits and/or hospitalizations

---

1. Institute of Medicine and National Resource Council, *From Cancer Patient to Cancer Survivor: Lost in Transition*, 4.

- Details of your responses to medications, including any side effects and reactions
- Details about follow-up care. For example, how often should you go back to see the oncologist? What tests and scans are needed and how often?
- Information about possible future symptoms. For example, what are the signs of possible recurrence? Which ones should you watch for, and which ones will a doctor monitor?
- Details about which doctor you should call for what. For example, who can help with lingering side effects from cancer treatment? Who is your go-to doctor for other health issues?
- Resources for managing the long-term financial impact of cancer
- Resources for help with social, emotional, and psychological issues

There is an organization in Chicago called the American College of Surgeons that oversees the Commission on Cancer (CoC), "a consortium of professional organizations dedicated to improving survival and quality of life for cancer patients."[2] The CoC sets the standards for the delivery of cancer care in the United States. It reviews and accredits hundreds of hospitals across the country. The commission recommends and encourages that hospitals and cancer centers provide you with a survivor care plan when you complete treatment. The commission also requires its accredited centers to screen patients for distress and offer some form of patient navigation. You can check to see if your cancer center is CoC-accredited or find a CoC-accredited cancer center on its website at www.facs.org/search/cancer-programs.

As you enter this new phase of life beyond treatment, you might find yourself dealing with certain medical issues. Some will go away in time, but others may linger. Here are some of the most common symptoms, and tips for how to deal with them.[3]

---

2. American College of Surgeons, Commission on Cancer, accessed October 21, 2020, www.facs.org/quality-programs/cancer/coc.

3. Adapted from "Cancer Transitions," Cancer Support Community, accessed October 21, 2020, www.cancersupportcommunity.org/cancer-transitions.

FATIGUE

"The number one complaint of cancer survivors is Cancer-Related Fatigue (CRF) which can affect an individual's relationships, daily activities, and economic state."
—American Journal of Nursing

"Bone-weary" is how some people describe it. Often, fatigue will dissipate over time. With a gradual increase in exercise and better nutrition habits, you will regain energy.

In some cases, treatment for cancer can cause anemia, which can lead to fatigue. Anemia is a drop in the blood's oxygen-carrying components. A simple blood test can determine whether you have anemia and its cause (such as iron deficiency). Changes to your diet can help relieve anemia. If needed, medication may help.

Tips to Fight Fatigue

- Plan carefully to take advantage of your best times of day.
- Set consistent times for waking and sleeping.
- Cut back on, but don't cut out, favorite pastimes.
- Find chances to rest.
- Creatively change or adapt normal activities to fit your energy level.
- Accept fewer responsibilities or volunteer activities to enable more "free time" for rest.
- Ask for help and allow others to help you.

SLEEP CHANGES

Sleep problems affect many people after treatment. Getting the right amount of sleep can be a struggle. At one end of the spectrum is hypersomnia, which causes people to sleep ten hours or more at a time. At the other end is insomnia, the inability to get enough sleep to let you feel rested. Hypersomnia, insomnia, and increased nightmares can aggravate other side effects. Sleep troubles can interfere with your ability to handle and enjoy everyday activities.

Tips for Managing Hypersomnia

- Try to get exercise every day, preferably in the morning or early afternoon.
- Develop a routine to sleep and wake the same time every day. When it is time to get up, get out of bed.
- Engage in activities that you enjoy, which call for your full attention.
- Avoid eating foods that make you sleepy during the day.

Tips for Managing Insomnia

- Work with your doctor to address underlying sources of insomnia, such as pain, anxiety, or stimulating medication.
- Sleep and wake at the same time each day.
- Avoid caffeine, alcohol, and tobacco, especially at night.
- If you are hungry at bedtime, eat a light snack.
- If you are able, exercise regularly.
- Sleep in a quiet, dark room that is not too hot or cold.
- Start a bedtime ritual, such as reading or taking a bath, to signal to your body that it is time for sleep.
- Medications are sometimes used to treat insomnia in the short term and only when other treatments are ineffective.

Tips for Dealing with Nightmares

- Talk about the nightmares. Reach out to a trusted family member, friend, or therapist.
- Write in a diary or draw pictures to express the content or themes of the nightmares.
- Imagine alternative endings or story lines to the nightmares.
- During the daytime, talk with someone close about your fears and feelings.

COGNITIVE CHANGES

Cognitive changes are problems with thinking, including memory, concentration, and behavior. Some cancers, cancer treatments, and medications can cause cognitive changes. There are also causes that are not related to cancer. Cognitive changes can affect your ability to work or complete everyday tasks. It is very upsetting to realize that your cancer has been successfully treated, but as a result you don't think or remember as clearly as you once did.

Chemotherapy, radiation, and surgery do not always lead to cognitive changes, but it is important to know what to look for. When survivors experience slight changes in their ability to remember or concentrate well after receiving chemotherapy, they are experiencing something commonly referred to as "chemo brain." Symptoms of chemo brain may include:

- difficulty concentrating
- difficulty remembering things that occurred recently
- confusion
- inability to think clearly

Whether cognitive changes will improve or be permanent depends on their cause. Acute cognitive changes that occur because of certain medications often improve when you stop taking the medicine. Chronic changes are often not reversible but may be improved if the cause of the problems can be corrected.

If you notice changes in your thinking, memory, or behavior, keep a record of the problems that you are experiencing. Ask your family and friends to watch for additional problems. Make an appointment to talk to your health care team about these symptoms as soon as possible.

LYMPHEDEMA

Lymphedema is swelling in the arms, legs, or trunk that occurs from a buildup of lymph fluid. Lymph fluid carries cells that help fight infections and other diseases to the parts of our body where they are needed. Lymphedema stops the lymph fluid from flowing freely in your body and often causes prominent swelling. Watch for even a slight increase in size or swelling of the arms, hands, fingers, chest wall, trunk, or legs. Contact your doctor if you notice these symptoms.

People who have had the following procedures are at higher risk for lymphedema:

- removal of lymph nodes
- biopsy
- lumpectomy or mastectomy
- surgery that disrupts lymph flow in the groin or armpit (this may include surgery for prostate and gynecologic cancers, and melanoma)
- sentinel lymph node mapping procedures (use of dyes and radioactive substances to identify lymph nodes that contain tumor cells)

Other factors—such as being overweight, having diabetes, and taking certain medications like steroids—may also put a cancer survivor at risk for lymphedema.

Strategies to lower your risk of lymphedema, or, if it develops, prevent symptoms from getting worse include:

- When possible, avoid injections, finger sticks, blood pressure checks, or blood draws in the arm that might be at risk for lymphedema (the post-surgery side).
- Keep the skin of the at-risk limb clean and gently moisturized.
- Make sure the at-risk arm or leg gets proper circulation.
- Lift the at-risk arm above the heart occasionally.
- Select a lightweight prosthetic, if required.
- Wear only loose-fitting clothing and jewelry around the affected area.
- Avoid heavy lifting, rigorous movements, and excessive pressure on the affected limb.
- Establish a safe exercise program (if there is discomfort, elevate the affected limb).
- Avoid extreme temperature changes (e.g., saunas, hot tubs).
- Minimize chances of injury and infection (e.g., bruises, cuts, insect bites, scratches) to the affected limb.
- Take special precautions when traveling. Ask for guidance from a lymphedema specialist.

PAIN

Treatment for cancer—surgery, chemotherapy, radiation therapy, and targeted therapies—can cause pain and discomfort. Because cancer can also cause pain, cancer survivors can become especially distressed when they notice new or worsening pain. They must manage both the pain itself and the worry over what it might mean. This is why relief from pain must address fears as well.

Studies show that pain among cancer survivors is often not reported, recognized, or treated well. Pain can keep you from living your life as fully as possible. But you do not have to suffer in silence. In most cases, treatment can help.

If you begin experiencing new pain or severe pain, tell your doctor immediately. When you talk with your doctor, they may ask you questions about the pain. They will want to know how often you have pain and how much the pain hurts. Using a pain rating scale will help your doctor better understand your pain and provide an appropriate course of treatment.

The Pain Rating Scale[4]

0	1	2	3	4	5	6	7	8	9	10
No Pain					Medium Pain					Worst Pain Possible

When you have pain, use this scale to write down how much the pain hurts:

- 0 means you have no pain
- 1 to 5 means you have mild pain
- 6 to 9 means you have severe pain
- 10 means you have the worst pain possible

---

4. "Cancer Transitions," Cancer Support Community. This tool was supported by Cooperative Agreement Number U58/CCU623066-01 from the Centers for Disease Control and Prevention. Its contents are solely the responsibility of the authors and do not necessarily represent the official views of the Centers for Disease Control and Prevention.

In order to prepare for a conversation with your doctor, it is a good idea to keep track of where, when, and how the pain occurs. You can write down the answers to the following questions:

- Where does it hurt? What are the exact places? Does the pain stay there or radiate out?
- Was the onset sudden or gradual? Is the pain constant or does it come and go?
- What makes the pain worse and/or better?
- How does it affect your life? Does it interfere with your usual activities, such as working, household chores, exercise, eating, or socializing with family and friends?

Relief from pain may involve one or more of the following:

- prescription or nonprescription drugs
- exercise
- physical or occupational therapy
- complementary medicine such as meditation and acupuncture
- surgery or nerve blocks

To help relieve pain, your doctor may prescribe medication or alternative therapies, such as yoga or massage therapy. If you have questions or concerns about pain management, or about medicines to treat your pain, be sure to ask questions. It is important that you ask all your questions and are satisfied with the answers. There are options, so, just like with cancer treatment, be sure to choose the approach that is right for you.

NERVE DAMAGE OR NEUROPATHY

Nerve damage from treatment—also called neuropathy—can cause odd sensations such as tingling, pain, or numbness in your hands, arms, feet, or legs. This type of damage raises your risk of burns and falls. For example, if your sense of touch is impaired, you can scald your skin in the shower without realizing it. If your legs are numb, you are more likely to stumble.

If nerve damage is a problem for you, there are practical steps you can take to make your environment safer:

- Check water temperature.
- Be sure to use gloves and pot holders.
- Keep rooms, outside paths, and stairs well lit.
- Clear walkways and floors.
- Use nonskid mats in showers and bathtubs.
- Ask your doctor or nurse what actions make sense for you, at home and at work.

As you move from patient to survivor, you can take some control over this next chapter in your life. Ask for a survivor care plan and get answers to your questions about next steps. Establish a good follow-up plan. Keep in touch with your doctors about symptoms and concerns. Make plans for the future, and use this time as an opportunity to make important lifestyle changes that will contribute to your long-term wellness and quality of life.

"During my treatment for acute myeloid leukemia, the intense focus on the battle to overcome the disease consumed so much of my energy that surviving was just a goal somewhere in an uncertain future. It was only when that first battle ended that I found that survivorship is a battle in its own right."
—Andy, acute myeloid leukemia survivor

RESOURCES FOR SURVIVORSHIP CARE

Cancer Support Community's "Beyond Treatment"—Resources to address lifestyle and health concerns beyond treatment. www.cancersupportcommunity.org/beyond -treatment

Cancer Support Community's "Moving Beyond Treatment" webinar—An eighty-five-minute webinar on issues that matter most to cancer survivors. www.youtube.com /watch?time_continue=36&v=Imbonv40GsA&feature=emb_logo

Cancer Support Community's "Cancer Survivorship"—Support and resources for cancer survivors. www.cancersupportcommunity.org/cancer-survivorship

Cancer Support Community's "Survivorship Care Planning" webinar—A ninety-minute webinar on survivorship that includes questions and answers by people just like you. www.youtube.com/watch?v=t4jpnhKDnPQ&feature=emb_logo

Cancer Support Community's "Cancer Transitions"—A comprehensive program designed to give you the energy and ability to cope with life after treatment. www .cancersupportcommunity.org/cancer-transitions

CHAPTER 28

Managing Fear of Recurrence

Treatment is over. You are now a cancer survivor. As we discussed in chapter twenty-six, the transition from patient to survivor can be an emotional one. You've been through a life-altering experience. It turned your world upside down and interrupted life as you knew it.

Some people share that ending treatment and having a moment to finally exhale leads to a recognition of all they've been through. They are confronted with some overwhelming emotions they weren't expecting. These emotions may include:[1]

- relief that it is over.
- a sense of the unknown.
- cautious optimism.

---

1. "Cancer Transitions," Cancer Support Community, accessed October 22, 2020, www.cancer supportcommunity.org/cancer-transitions.

- anger or guilt about the cancer.
- fear that cancer will come back (recurrence).
- grief and loss for the old life or body.
- concerns about living with cancer.
- discomfort or shame about needing help with a chronic illness.
- uncertainty about what to do next.
- frustration with physical changes.

You may experience one or more of these emotions as the reality of treatment ending sinks in. Starting to look to the future may feel a little scary or confusing. The plans you once had may not fit anymore.

Central to your thoughts may be a concern shared by many cancer survivors: Will the cancer return? This is often called fear of recurrence. For some, these fears can be debilitating. They may consume your thoughts. It might feel like the worry is taking over your life. When you are not feeling well, are fatigued, or have a new ache or pain, your first thought may be, *I wonder if the cancer is back*. Your fears may come to the surface if you take follow-up medicine for your cancer. A pill can become a daily reminder of your cancer experience. The anniversary of a cancer diagnosis can bring fear or worry. Some people also have elevated anxiety when they get close to the date of scans and other follow-up tests. This is sometimes called "scanxiety."

As fear of recurrence bubbles up, consider these tips that can help you regain control and manage those fears:

Tips for Coping with Fear of Recurrence[2]

- Learn the signs for recurrence of your type of cancer.
- Keep up with any medical tests or appointments your doctor recommends.
- Talk about it—express your feelings.
- You do not have to be upbeat all the time, but look for the positive.
- Be empowered—take control of what you can, make a plan, and know what you cannot control.

---

2. "Cancer Transitions," Cancer Support Community.

One of the most important things you can do to care for yourself is to pay attention. Listen to the narrative in your head. Look at what you are and are not doing. Try to avoid making choices that are not ultimately in your own best interest.

People sometimes put off follow-up appointments and scans because of the emotions they can bring up. But avoiding these appointments may only elevate your risk for cancer recurrence. Close medical monitoring is key. By remaining diligent with follow-up care, you can take some control over your future. While no one can guarantee that the cancer won't return, having a good plan in place and keeping your follow-up appointments will help reduce your risk.

When you feel the fear of recurrence start to take over, use the exercise in the following guest essay by Maria Fanelli to help manage the fear and reduce your anxiety.

If you find your emotions after cancer treatment are unmanageable, or beyond what you can handle, seek help. Refer back to chapters eighteen and twenty-one, on emotional support and mind-body techniques, respectively. The same strategies you used to cope with treatment may help you now. Consider looking for a support group for cancer survivors or talk to your doctor. There are medications and other techniques that can help with anxiety and aid your path to recovery and wellness.

Easing the Fear of Recurrence:
A Meditation with Affirmations

MARIA FANELLI, LLC

Maria Fanelli is a seasoned mindfulness instructor, life coach, and mind-body health educator who teaches clients how to clarify and cultivate a forward path to their goals.

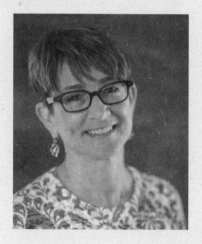

Fear of cancer recurrence is a normal, yet sometimes terrifying, reaction to a thought about the possibility of cancer returning. When we have this type of experience, it is due to what is known as a "fight or flight" reaction. This is when the brain is trying to keep the body safe from a threat by signaling to the body via hormones/adrenalin, to either run from the threat or to fight it. It is an antiquated trigger that has been carried over in this modern age from thousands of years ago, as far back as the time of cavemen and women and saber-toothed tigers.

We can easily recognize this automatic reaction when we feel a surge of fear-based energy in the body such as blood pressure rising, our heart beating rapidly, sudden perspiration, tensing muscles, etc. The vast majority of the time we do not need this intense reaction! Many times, we are in a safe place with no immediate threat whatsoever! However, one little thought may arise that scares us and then this type of reaction happens instantly. The fear reaction is typically superheightened and it continues to build, fueled by more and more scary thoughts that continue to increase the sense of fear in our body even more. While in this propelled fear state, we are not mentally, emotionally, or physically balanced at all. We are completely lost in fear thoughts that are triggering intense physical sensations and emotions. It doesn't matter if they are realistic or imagined or if they are based on any evidence—the feeling is the same and it can feel very turbulent and uncomfortable.

The good news is that we can calm it. Below is a five-step meditation/affirmation process to use any time you feel fear of recurrence:

1. STOP THE CYCLE!

The first thing to do is to stop fueling the fear cycle. Wherever you are, start by bringing your attention to focusing on taking a nice deeper breath. Then take another one and this time put your hand on your chest or abdomen. Keep your hand in place as it will help to keep you grounded. Begin to feel your hand and body moving with the breath. Continue to follow the breath and movement with your attention—the full in-breath and the full out-breath. Breathing in, breathing out. Do this for a few breaths. You have now stopped the cycle!

2. FIND FEAR IN YOUR BODY.

The next piece is to actually feel into the torso to see if you can notice where the fear actually is. Be curious about it. Where is this fear? It may feel like a lot of energy in one area, or feel like a heavy weight, or it may feel totally different for you. Once you locate it, give it a number of intensity from 1 to 10. How strong is it? Notice what it is actually doing. Observe the characteristics of it—is it hot, is it cold, is it vibrating, does it feel jagged or smooth, is it big or small, is it heavy or light? What do you notice? Continue to stay steady with the breath as you explore this area. Breathing in and out, nice and easy.

3. ACCEPT THESE SENSATIONS.

Once you recognize the sensations of fear in the body, welcome them to be here. Accept that you are experiencing whatever sensations are present and just acknowledge them. Chances are they will not want to stay once you welcome them, but if you try to get rid of them or hold them down or push them away, or run away from these sensations, they most likely will want to stay. So, welcome and accept the feelings of fear that you notice. Fear is not you. Fear is just an emotion with body sensations that we label as fear. Fear is a feeling and probably a very familiar one for you. If so, it may help to call it your old friend, fear. "Here it is again, my old friend, fear." Remember, it is the emotion your body creates when the brain and body automatically react to a real or perceived threat. This can be a real threat or just a passing and possibly imagined thought. Sometimes, it may build up so much that it turns into a future catastrophic movie! However, the body does not know the difference between something that is real and something we are imagining and therefore the reaction is the same. The good news is that the brain is doing its job to alert you of a possible threat, even though you probably do not need to be alerted! For now, welcome the body sensations and emotion of fear. Sometimes they just need a little attention to settle down. You are still breathing in and breathing out and staying anchored with the breath.

4. TELL YOURSELF AND YOUR BODY WHAT YOU WANT THEM TO KNOW.

Your body listens to you. Our thoughts talk to our cells. Remind yourself that you will get through whatever comes up. Give your cells some confidence. You have already faced so much and are so brave and courageous that you will be able to face whatever shows up when it shows up, *if* it shows up. You do not need to imagine something now that may or may not ever happen. Now close your eyes and use your imagination to picture yourself hugging a young child or someone you care about. You are reassuring them that everything will be okay. You are giving them a big hug and they are feeling safe and comfortable and loved. Then with this same feeling you have in giving this person a hug, give this hug to yourself. You're feeling safe, comfortable, loved, and proud of yourself. And thank your body for what a good job it *is* doing. Focus on all the good that is actually happening. Notice all the positive things your body is able to do—remind yourself of all the things your body is doing well right now... Remember that your body is constantly generating new healthy cells and all these positive thoughts and feelings are boosting those healthy cells even more. Know that there is much more right with you than wrong with you. Bring to mind all the areas in your life that are working well. All the things you are so grateful for. And then send yourself some healing affirmations:

- I love and accept myself, just I am.
- I am good enough, just as I am.
- I love every part of myself and all my uniqueness.
- Thank you, cells, for doing an amazing job.
- Thank you, brain, for always trying to keep me safe.
- Thank you, organs and tissues, for working hard and doing miraculous things to keep me healthy.
- Thank you to me for taking care of myself, just like I am doing right now.
- May I be more patient and kind to myself, every day.

Breathing in, breathing out.

5. BE PRESENT.

If you moved your hand from your stomach or chest, gently bring it back. Feel yourself breathing here and allow the body to open to the breath so you feel it flowing into and out of the body. Notice any sensations that are present, even noticing if some fear is still present. If so, see if the intensity has changed from before when you gave it a number from 1 to 10. What number is it now? Once again, bring the focus of your attention to feeling the body moving as you breathe in and breathe out. Nice and easy. Breathing in and breathing out. Then notice how in this exact moment, with this exact breath, that everything is okay. When thoughts arise, just gently, yet firmly, come back to feeling the body moving with the breath. Feel your hand on the body, feel the body steady in this moment. In this moment, all is well. In this moment, you are accepting your body just as it is. Your body is loved. You are loved. You are present. Allow yourself to be present in this moment and know that you can always connect to this space, to this presence. It never leaves you. Now allow this greater sense of well-being to expand all throughout your body and even outside your body. And when you are ready, proceed with this grounded presence into the next moment.

RESOURCES FOR COPING WITH FEAR OF RECURRENCE

Cancer.net's "Coping with Fear of Recurrence"—Advice for coping with fear of recurrence from the American Society of Clinical Oncology. www.cancer.net/survivorship/life-after-cancer/coping-with-fear-recurrence

Cancer Support Community's "Cancer Transitions"—A comprehensive program designed to give you the energy and ability to cope with life after treatment. www.cancersupportcommunity.org/cancer-transitions

Cancer Support Community's "How to Manage Fear of Cancer Recurrence"—www.cancersupportcommunity.org/blog/2018/02/how-manage-fear-cancer-recurrence

CHAPTER 29

Hospice and End of Life

There may come a time when cancer treatment stops working and there are no other treatment options available. This is sometimes called *terminal disease*. This news can be incredibly difficult to process, both for the person with cancer and for their loved ones. It can bring with it a wide range of emotions, including anger, fear, sadness, depression, and eventually, acceptance.

If you have come to this point, you may find it challenging to manage your fears and anxieties. Some people in this situation have found it helpful to acknowledge and name their fears in order to deal with them. Here are some thoughts on how to do that:

Acknowledge Your Specific Fears[1]

- *Fear of the unknown:* It is normal to be afraid of the things we can't imagine. If you have been involved in a faith community or other spiritual group, you may find some answers there that will be helpful to you.

- *Fear of pain and suffering:* Many people fear that pain and suffering at the end of life cannot be avoided. Talking with your health care team about your concerns is very important. They will help you understand the advances in medicine that can minimize pain and lessen anxiety and depression.

- *Fear of punishment:* People with religious beliefs and those with no religion at all may fear that they will be punished for what they did or did not do. Each of us has things we would do differently if we could go back in time. Sharing your regrets openly with those close to you or with someone from a faith community can help you feel less burdened.

- *Worry about what will happen to your loved ones:* Most people worry about what will happen to those who are dependent on them. Making plans in advance for guardianship and finances can help lessen these kinds of worries.

- *Worry about loss of control:* It is our nature to want to be in control over our lives, but recognizing what is out of our control can help us focus attention on the things we can control.

- *Fear of isolation:* Being open about what you are really thinking and feeling with those close to you will help them feel more comfortable being around you. Let them know that you still want to know what is happening in their lives and that it is okay to joke and talk about trivial things as well as discussing some of the more serious things on their minds.

- *Fear of nonexistence:* Many people, including those who are not religious, believe in the afterlife. When facing death, it is not unusual to question this belief. We cannot know for sure what will happen, but you may find it reassuring to talk about this with others in your faith community or with your loved ones.

---

1. "Managing Fear," Cancer Support Community, accessed October 22, 2020, www.cancer supportcommunity.org/managing-fear.

As you acknowledge and work to address your fears, you may also want to think about things you can do to find a sense of closure—to feel more at peace. This may mean healing a broken relationship, expressing your true feelings about something or someone, or accepting that life will go on without you. This is also a moment in life when you may want to turn to a member of a faith community, counselor, or therapist. This person can help you talk through your concerns, acknowledge them, and find healing and peace.

Some patients decide to end treatment but feel reluctant to share their decision with their family or their doctor. They worry that their family will feel that they are giving up or that their doctor might think they are not a fighter. A patient in Philadelphia once told me that instead of telling his family he was giving up, he told them he was letting go—letting go of the pain, the suffering, the endless treatments, and the disappointment. He was ready to move on to this next chapter, even though he knew it was his final chapter.

If you are starting to write your final chapter, think about how you are going to find physical and emotional comfort. The next two sections address important ways you can care for yourself and others during this time.

HOSPICE

When treatment ends, it is time to think about hospice care. Hospice is a specialized area of health care that focuses on end of life. Hospice addresses a breadth of needs, ranging from relief from pain and other symptoms to the emotional and spiritual issues people cope with at the end of life. It is important to distinguish hospice from palliative care. Palliative care is a medical specialty focused on symptom management. It is appropriate for any stage of cancer, at any point in treatment. Hospice is just for end of life. It is generally considered when someone is thought to have less than six months to live.

When we think about hospice, we often imagine a person with only days to live, but that is usually not the case. In many instances, a person is in hospice care for weeks or even months. Hospice can be a meaningful part of this time of life. People in hospice sometimes find it easier to make their wishes known and seek closure.

If you are considering ending treatment, call a hospice program to explore your options. Find out how it can help. Hospice care can be provided at home or at a special hospice care facility. Look into the types of hospice services that are available in your community. The right approach for you will depend on your needs and the level of support being provided by family and friends. As you make plans, find out what your insurance will cover. Planning in advance can create a smoother transition.

QUESTIONS TO ASK YOUR INSURANCE COMPANY ABOUT HOME HEALTH CARE AND HOSPICE CARE[2]

- Do I have a home health care benefit? If so, what does it cover? Is there a maximum number of covered visits?
- Are there co-pays associated with home health care visits?
- Do I have a home or inpatient hospice benefit? What does it cover? Is it separate from my home health benefit? Is there a lifetime cap of covered services?
- What is the best way to utilize both of these benefits?
- Will there be a co-pay for each individual home health or home hospice visit?
- Do I have to use a preferred provider? If so, who are the preferred providers?
- To ensure coverage, does my health insurance company need to pre-approve home or inpatient hospice care before it is started?
- What are my alternatives to home health or home hospice care?
- I have a long-term care insurance plan that covers home health care. How do I access these benefits?

---

2. Cancer Support Community, *Frankly Speaking About Cancer: Coping with the Cost of Care*, March 2020, www.cancersupportcommunity.org/managing-cost -cancer-treatment.

People are sometimes wary of hospice. Keep in mind that hospice is there to support you. The focus is on improving your quality of life and decreasing your pain and suffering. Hospice can also provide valuable support to your loved ones, offering them both respite and the assurance that you will be treated with respect and your wishes will be honored.

FINDING CLOSURE AND LEAVING A LEGACY

In addition to making plans for your medical care at end of life, you also want to look for ways to find closure. You may do this by talking with loved ones and telling them how you feel. You may want to thank people who have supported you or reach out to those who have been absent from your life for a long time. For some, this can be a time to apologize to those they have hurt.

You may also start to think about your legacy. Legacy has different meanings, but people often focus on the wishes, lessons, values, or memories they want to leave behind for their loved ones. You can approach this in many ways.

Some people choose to prepare an ethical will. While a standard will is a legal document that outlines the distribution of worldly possessions, like cash or real estate, an ethical will lays out the values you want to leave behind for your loved ones. This is a chance to consider the values that have steered your life—like family, responsibility, generosity, equality, faith, quest for knowledge, or others. Parents, especially, may find this a meaningful way to reflect on their life and share what they have learned.

Perhaps your focus is more on the future and the life events you will miss. Or just simple thoughts to share. As you start to think about your legacy, you may want to gather mementos or create messages. They may include:

Family photos: Some people like to take time to sort through family photos to organize them and create captions or notes about the people and the places pictured.

Videos: You may want to tell stories on video about special moments or times in your life, like your childhood memories, how you met your spouse, or a special vacation. Videos can also include stories about your work or your hobbies—and things that you did to improve your community or society as a whole. Or you may want to describe hard times and the struggles you faced.

Recipes: Perhaps you have some favorite recipes that your friends and family enjoy and always look forward to. Write these recipes down. Your loved ones will think of you when they make these dishes, and that will evoke fond memories of your time together.

Notes for the future: Knowing that they may not be here to celebrate important milestones for family and loved ones in the future, some people like to write cards, notes, or letters to be given to their loved ones on a significant birthday, graduation, or wedding day. Even though you may not be here to celebrate those moments, your loved ones will know you are with them and will cherish your expressions of love and support. You can also record video or audio to be shared at certain times.

Other items of importance: While you are still living, you may want to give items of sentimental value to loved ones and share the stories of why these things are important. It could be a childhood toy, an item of clothing, or a knickknack that has meaning or a special memory attached.

Regardless of how you choose to leave your legacy, know that your life had meaning. The memories of your contributions and life lessons imparted will endure.

Most importantly at this time of life, be gentle with yourself. Take care of yourself. Lean on others and seek help as needed. Spend time with people and on activities that bring you joy. Make the most of these days. The journey is not over yet.

Grief Connects Us

JOSEPH STERN, MD

Joseph Stern, MD (josephsternmd.com), is the author of Grief Connects Us: A Neurosurgeon's Lessons on Love, Loss, and Compassion *(Central Recovery Press). He is a partner in the country's largest neurosurgical group practice, Carolina Neurosurgery and Spine Associates, and practices general adult neurosurgery at the Moses H. Cone Hospital, the flagship hospital of Cone Health in Greensboro, North Carolina.*

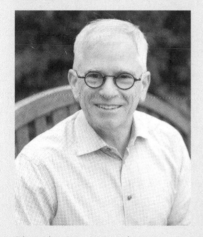

Photo by Aura Marzouk

I used to keep my distance from patients. I explained things thoroughly, but often with a courtesy based in fear: technically correct, yet detached.

Two experiences reshaped my appreciation of the liberating powers of grief and compassion. My sister Victoria developed leukemia, had a bone marrow transplant, and died. Eighteen months later, her husband, Pat, had a brain hemorrhage from which he lapsed into a coma. After brain surgery and a two-week hospitalization without improvement, we withdrew treatment. Pat also died, leaving their teenage sons parentless.

Now, I let my patients and their families know I care. I pull them close when things are going badly and acknowledge their suffering. I have opened up to the power of solace, gratitude, and compassion, and to an understanding of the fear and isolation that come with their absence. I try to keep that window open for others.

I have come to accept that I am powerless to fix problems or cure illnesses in patients I desperately want to help. With his mother, I stood at the bedside of a young man. He had been paralyzed in a devastating car accident and was about to die. There was nothing we could do to save him. Words failed me. Instead of pulling back, I reached out to her and hugged her. We held onto each other and cried. I couldn't help her son. But I did something to help her. And she helped me in return.

Victoria's illness and death broke down the protective barriers I had built over my career. Despite all our knowledge and skill, we are frequently powerless to undo that which has befallen us. Physicians must cure when we can and console when we cannot, while being as honest and empathetic as possible. We must be willing to recognize our limitations and to accept defeat. Avoiding the connected emotions of grief and compassion doesn't just fail to protect us: it is corrosive.

With the coronavirus pandemic, grief and loss have affected us all. As I told a dear friend on the accidental death of his teenage son, who died at the height of the pandemic: grief connects us with our better selves. While transformative, the process of grieving is painful and disruptive: I wouldn't wish it on anyone. Once through it, there's also no going back.

We have these experiences as individuals; they define the human condition. With the pandemic, they are shared, even as the losses we feel during this time are magnified in their intensity because the rituals we rely on to mark the transitions of our lives are disallowed. Weddings and graduations have been canceled; births and deaths unattended. My friend's family was unable to have a funeral, just as others have died alone and been buried without celebration.

Working through our personal grief is restorative, but now we can experience collective grief as a uniting force. Shared grief connects us more closely with each other, leading us toward compassion, gratitude, and grace.

RESOURCES FOR HOSPICE AND END OF LIFE

Cancer Support Community's "Bereavement"—Covers topics such as facing loss, finding acceptance, and taking care of yourself. www.cancersupportcommunity.org /bereavement

Cancer Support Community's "Caregivers"—Support and resources for caregivers of people with cancer. www.cancersupportcommunity.org/caregivers

Cancer Support Community's "On Your Terms: A Conversation About End-of-Life Care"—An hour-long episode of the Cancer Support Community's weekly radio broadcast focused on end of life. www.cancersupportcommunity.org/radio-show /your-terms-conversation-about-end-life-care

Hospice Foundation—A comprehensive resource on understanding, choosing, preparing for, and paying for hospice. hospicefoundation.org/Hospice-Care

National Hospice and Palliative Care Organization (NHPCO)—Information on hospice, caregivers, advance directives, and more. www.nhpco.org/patients-and-caregivers

ACKNOWLEDGMENTS

This book represents the wisdom, toil, and inspiration of so many people. It is difficult to list them all, but I will do my very best.

First and most importantly, I want to thank all the patients and caregivers who have shared their stories with us, trusted us when they were most vulnerable, and inspired us with their grace and indomitable spirit.

Next, I would like to thank the Cancer Support Community (CSC), where I have spent the past twenty-plus years of my career. I have worked with extraordinary, smart, and passionate staff, board, affiliate leaders, volunteers, donors, advisers, and partners to advance the idea that community is stronger than cancer and to ensure that no one faces cancer alone. CSC has nurtured me, supported me, been patient with me, and entertained many of my unorthodox and sometimes far-fetched ideas over the years! Thank you for trusting me and fostering my spirit and enthusiasm.

A special and heartfelt thank-you to the amazing CSC staff and leadership team, and the executive team, including Linda Bohannon, Elizabeth Franklin, and Jeff Travers. You are my Team One. And a deep and sincere expression of gratitude to our entire board of directors, including the executive committee: Lauren Barnes, Jill Durovsik, Lynne O'Brien, Andy Sandler, and Holly Tyson. You are always there when it matters most.

There are several staff members at CSC who were a critical part of this project, and I want to acknowledge their invaluable contributions. Nathalie Casthely is this book's protective aunt, its shepherd, and its guiding light. Ted Miller brings the "big picture" perspective to this project and a special finesse to all we do. He will make sure the book reaches those who need it most. Claire Saxton oversees our Education Department and "Frankly Speaking" series and was the tireless champion who curated the incredible, rich, high-quality "Frankly Speaking" content contained herein. That thank-you also extends to the incredible medical professionals, writers, researchers, editors, interns, designers, photographers, and contractors who, over the years, have helped us write, edit, improve, and update our educational materials. You know who you are. Thank you also to Susan Ash-Lee, Karen Costello, and Sally Werner for their support on this project and for their incredible work on behalf of patients and families.

Thank you to the wonderful friends and champions of our mission who contributed essays and quotes in support of the project. A special Philly thank-you to Jill Biden, who is a true advocate for all those impacted by cancer. She always speaks from the heart and manages to reach into a person's soul and touch and inspire them in a profound way. Cancer patients and their loved ones are in a better place because she has their backs.

I would also like to thank the team at BenBella Books for believing in this project and taking such good care with it. I know you are passionate about the subject matter and share our commitment to ensuring that this resource reaches as many people touched by cancer as possible.

I owe a very special debt of gratitude to my "wing woman" on this project, Jamie Kudera. Jamie was my researcher and editor, but more than that, she poured herself into making this book better every step of the way. We discovered through this project that we actually went to high school together at the Philadelphia High School for Girls. How fortuitous that we came back together all these years later for such an important cause.

I wish all of you could meet the amazing Dr. Craig Cole. If you did, you would say, "Gosh, I wish he were *my* doctor!" He is kind, compassionate, patient, a good listener, and a great standard-bearer for patient-centered care. He brought his keen medical mind to this project and kept us honest every step of the way.

A special and very personal thank-you to my amazing, smart, curious, funny friends, who laugh at my jokes, listen to my endless travel stories, and inspire me to be a better person.

And last, but not least, a warm and heartfelt thank-you to my family for always sticking by me—even though we don't always agree. Thank you, Mom and Dad, Joann and Bert, for encouraging me to pursue my dreams, even though they didn't always make sense to you. Thank you to my siblings and siblings-in-law: Mark, Julie, Kristina, David, Matthew, and Andrew. And to my nieces and nephews: Mark, Nija, Kaelin, Paige, Adam, JoHannah, Maura, David, Chloe, and Claire—you are my true muses. To all of you I say be kind, be curious, be a good friend, stand up for those who don't have a voice, laugh a lot, see the world, give people the benefit of the doubt, and try to find small ways to make a difference.

CANCER SUPPORT COMMUNITY BOARD OF DIRECTORS

CANCER SUPPORT COMMUNITY PROFESSIONAL ADVISORY BOARD

Barry Bultz, PhD | The University of Calgary, psychologist

Stephanie Cohen, MS, LCGC | St. Vincent Health, genetic counselor

Sanja Dacic, MD, PhD | University of Pittsburgh Medical Center, director of pathology

Christina M. Dieli-Conwright, PhD, MD, FACSM | Dana-Farber Cancer Institute, Harvard Medical School, physiologist

Bruce Edelen | Oncology Reimbursement Management Inc., oncology reimbursement specialist

Stephen Edge, MD | Roswell Park Comprehensive Cancer Center, surgical oncologist

Henry Friedman, MD | Duke University School of Medicine, brain cancer specialist

Mary Lou Galantino, PT, MS, PhD, MSCE, FNAP, FAPTA | Stockton University, rehabilitation specialist

Ashley Haggerty, MD, MSCE | University of Pennsylvania Perelman School of Medicine, GYN cancers specialist

Karen Hurley, PhD | The Cleveland Clinic, clinical psychologist and patient advocate

Rupesh Kotecha, MD | Miami Cancer Institute, radiation oncologist

Thomas LeBlanc, MD | Duke University School of Medicine, blood cancers specialist

Sharyn Lewin, MD | Holy Name Medical Center, GYN cancers specialist

CANCER SUPPORT COMMUNITY AFFILIATES

U.S. Affiliates

ARIZONA

CSC ARIZONA
Phoenix, AZ
Phone: 602-712-1006
www.cscaz.org

CALIFORNIA

CSC CALIFORNIA CENTRAL COAST
Templeton, CA 93465
Phone: 805-238-4411
www.cscslo.org

**CSC LOS ANGELES
THE BENJAMIN CENTER**
Los Angeles, CA
Phone: 310-314-2555
www.cancersupportla.org

CSC PASADENA
Pasadena, CA
Phone: 626-796-1083
www.cscpasadena.org

CSC REDONDO BEACH
Redondo Beach, CA
Phone: 310-376-3550
www.cancersupportredondobeach.org

CSC SAN FRANCISCO BAY AREA
Walnut Creek, CA
Phone: 925-933-0107
www.cancersupport.net

CSC VALLEY / VENTURA / SANTA BARBARA
Westlake Village, CA
Phone: 805-379-4777
www.cancersupportvvsb.org

COLORADO

CSC SOUTHWEST COLORADO
*Affiliate in development
Durango, CO 81302
Phone: 970-403-3711
www.blueprintsofhope.org

DELAWARE

CSC DELAWARE
Wilmington, DE
Phone: 302-995-2850
www.cancersupportdelaware.org

FLORIDA

GC SOUTH FLORIDA
Fort Lauderdale, FL
Phone: 954-763-6776
www.gildasclubsouthflorida.org

GEORGIA

CSC ATLANTA
Atlanta, GA
Phone: 404-843-1880
www.cscatlanta.org

ILLINOIS

GC CHICAGO
Chicago, IL
Phone: 312-464-9900
www.gildasclubchicago.org

INDIANA

CSC CENTRAL INDIANA
Indianapolis, IN
Phone: 317-257-1505
www.cancersupportindy.org

GC EVANSVILLE
Evansville, IN
Phone: 812-402-8667
www.gcevv.org

IOWA

GC QUAD CITIES
Davenport, IA
Phone: 563-326-7504
www.gildasclubqc.org

KENTUCKY

GC KENTUCKIANA
Louisville, KY 40204
Phone: 502-583-0075
www.gck.org

MICHIGAN

CSC GREATER ANN ARBOR
Ann Arbor, MI
Phone: 734-975-2500
www.cancersupportannarbor.org

GC GRAND RAPIDS
Grand Rapids, MI
Phone: 616-453-8300
www.gildasclubgr.org

GC METRO DETROIT
Royal Oak, MI
Phone: 248-577-0800
www.gildasclubdetroit.org

MINNESOTA

GC TWIN CITIES
Minnetonka, MN
Phone: 612-227-2147
www.gildasclubtwincities.org

MISSOURI

CSC GREATER ST. LOUIS
St. Louis, MO
Phone: 314-238-2000
www.cancersupportstl.org

GC KANSAS CITY
Kansas City, MO
Phone: 816-531-5444
www.gildasclubkc.org

MONTANA

CSC MONTANA
Bozeman, MT 59715
Phone: 406-582-1600
cancersupportmontana.org

NEW HAMPSHIRE

GC NEW HAMPSHIRE
*Affiliate in development
Laconia, NH 03246
Phone: 603-387-6775
www.gildasclubnh.org

NEW JERSEY

GC SOUTH JERSEY
Linwood, NJ
Phone: 609-926-2699
www.gildasclubsouthjersey.org

NEW YORK

GC ROCHESTER
Rochester, NY
Phone: 585-423-9700
www.gildasclubrochester.org

GC WESTCHESTER
White Plains, NY
Phone: 914-644-8844
www.gildasclubwestchester.org

OHIO

CSC CENTRAL OHIO
Columbus, OH
Phone: 614-884-4673
www.cancersupportohio.org

**CSC GREATER CINCINNATI–
NORTHERN KENTUCKY**
Cincinnati, OH
Phone: 513-791-4060
www.mycancersupportcommunity.org

PENNSYLVANIA

CSC GREATER LEHIGH VALLEY
Allentown, PA
Phone: 610-861-7555
www.cancersupportglv.org

CSC GREATER PHILADELPHIA
The Suzanne Morgan Center at
Ridgeland
Philadelphia, PA
Phone: 215-879-7733
www.cancersupportphiladelphia.org

TENNESSEE

CSC CHATTANOOGA
*Affiliate in development
Chattanooga, TN 37408

CSC EAST TENNESSEE
Knoxville, TN
Phone: 865-546-4661
www.CancerSupportet.org

GC MEMPHIS
*Affiliate in development
Germantown, TN 38183-0552
Phone: 901-833-1543
 www.gildasclubmemphis.org

GC MIDDLE TENNESSEE
Nashville, TN
Phone: 615-329-1124
www.gildasclubmiddletn.org

TEXAS

CSC NORTH TEXAS
Dallas, TX
Phone: 214-345-8230
www.cancersupporttexas.org

WASHINGTON, DC

CSC Washington, DC
*Affiliate in development
Phone: 202-650-5364
www.cancersupportcommunity.org/
WashingtonDC

WISCONSIN

GC MADISON
Middleton, WI
Phone: 608-828-8880
www.gildasclubmadison.org

International Affiliates

CANADA

GC GREATER TORONTO
Toronto, Ontario, Canada
Phone: 416-214-9898
www.gildasclubtoronto.org

**GC SIMCOE MUSKOKA
(Formerly Barrie, Ontario)**
Barrie, Ontario, Canada
Phone: 705-726-5199
www.gildasclubsimcoemuskoka.org

ISRAEL

TWC TEL AVIV
(Beit Mati)
Givatayim, Israel
Phone: 972-3-572-1630
www.cancer.org.il

JAPAN

CSC JAPAN
Cancer Support Community
Toranomon, Minato-ku
Tokyo, Japan
Phone: 81-3-5545-1805
www.csc-japan.org

Health Care Partners

ARIZONA

**TUBA CITY REGIONAL HEALTH
CARE**
Tuba City, AZ
www.tchealth.org

COLORADO

**ROCKY MOUNTAIN CANCER
CENTERS**
Lone Tree, CO
Phone: 303-925-0700
www.rockymountaincancercenters.com/
places/lone-tree/lone-tree-skyridge/

CONNECTICUT

**HARTFORD HEALTHCARE
CANCER INSTITUTE**
Hartford, CT 06102
Phone: 860-972-3086
https://hartfordhealthcare.org/services/
cancer-care

FLORIDA

**UF HEALTH CANCER CENTER–
ORLANDO HEALTH**
Orlando, FL 32806
Phone: 321-841-5056
www.ufhealthcancerorlando.com/
our-services/integrative-medicine

HAWAII

KONA COMMUNITY HOSPITAL
Kealakekua, HI 96750
Phone: 808-332-6910
www.kch.hhsc.org

MICHIGAN

**CSC AT INDIAN FAMILY HEALTH
CLINIC-GREAT FALLS**
Great Falls, MT 59401
Phone: 406-268-1510
www.ifhcgf.org

MISSOURI

MOSAIC LIFE CARE
St. Joseph, MO
Phone: 816-271-7657
www.mymosaiclifecare.org

NEW JERSEY

HOLY NAME MEDICAL CENTER
Teaneck, NJ
Phone: 201-833-3392
www.holyname.org

MONMOUTH MEDICAL CENTER (MONMOUTH COUNTY)
Long Branch, NJ
Phone: 732-923-6090
www.rwjbh.org/
monmouth-medical-center

MONMOUTH MEDICAL CENTER SOUTHERN CAMPUS (OCEAN COUNTY)
Lakewood, NJ
Phone: 732-923-6090
www.rwjbh.org/monmouth-medical
-center-southern-campus

PENNSYLVANIA
GETTYSBURG CANCER CENTER
Gettysburg, PA 17325
Phone: 717-337-5991 ext. 330
www.gettysburgcancercenter.com

SOUTH CAROLINA
PRISMA HEALTH CANCER INSTITUTE
Greenville, SC
Phone: 864-455-5809
www.ghs.org

WASHINGTON
NORTHWEST MEDICAL SPECIALTIES
Puyallup, WA
253-428-8700
www.nwmedicalspecialties.com

WASHINGTON, DC
WHITMAN-WALKER HEALTH CLINIC
Washington, DC 20009
Phone: 202-745-7000
www.whitman-walker.org

CANCER PATIENT ADVOCACY GROUPS AND RESOURCES

African American Breast Cancer Alliance

aabcainc.org

Educates and supports African Americans in their journeys with breast cancer and survivorship.

AIM at Melanoma

www.aimatmelanoma.org

Advances the battle against melanoma through innovative research, legislative reform, education, and patient and caregiver support.

American Brain Tumor Association

www.abta.org

Advances the understanding and treatment of brain tumors with the goals of improving, extending, and, ultimately, saving the lives of those impacted by a brain tumor diagnosis.

American Cancer Society (ACS)

www.cancer.org

ACS's mission is to save lives, celebrate lives, and lead the fight for a world without cancer.

American Cancer Society Cancer Action Network (ACS CAN)

www.fightcancer.org

An organization empowering volunteers to influence political change and impact the future of cancer.

American Childhood Cancer Organization
www.acco.org
A community of families, survivors, and friends who have been affected by childhood and adolescent cancer. Offers support, information, and advocacy.

American Liver Foundation
www.liverfoundation.org
Facilitates, advocates, and promotes education, support, and research for the prevention, treatment, and cure of liver disease.

American Lung Association (ALA)
www.lung.org
Saves lives by improving lung health and preventing lung disease through research, education, and advocacy.

Bladder Cancer Advocacy Network (BCAN)
www.bcan.org
A community of patients, caregivers, survivors, advocates, medical, and research professionals united in support of people touched by bladder cancer.

Blue Faery: The Adrienne Wilson Liver Cancer Association
www.bluefaery.org
Aims to prevent, treat, and cure primary liver cancer, specifically hepatocellular carcinoma, through research, education, and advocacy.

Brain Tumor Foundation
www.braintumorfoundation.org
Guides and supports patients and families during the turbulent times following the diagnosis of a brain tumor.

BreastCancer.org
www.breastcancer.org
Helps women, men, and their loved ones make sense of the complex medical and personal information about breast health and breast cancer so they can make the best decisions for their lives.

BreastCancerTrials.org

www.breastcancertrials.org

Encourages individuals affected by breast cancer to consider clinical trials as a routine option for care.

Bright Pink

www.brightpink.org

Saves lives from breast and ovarian cancer by empowering women to know their risk and manage their health proactively.

Cancer + Careers

www.cancerandcareers.org

Empowers and educates people with cancer to thrive in their workplace, by providing expert advice, interactive tools, and educational events.

CancerCare

www.cancercare.org

Provides free, professional support services, including counseling, support groups, educational workshops, publications, and financial assistance, to anyone affected by cancer.

Cancer Legal Resource Center

thedrlc.org/cancer/

Provides invaluable cancer-related legal information and resources to people nationwide.

Caregiver Action Network

caregiveraction.org

Promotes resourcefulness and respect for the more than ninety million family caregivers across the country.

Clearity Foundation

www.clearityfoundation.org

Strives to improve the survival and quality of life of women with ovarian cancer.

CLL Society

cllsociety.org

Focuses on patient education, support, and research to address the unmet needs of the chronic lymphocytic leukemia (CLL) and related blood cancer communities.

Coalition for Clinical Trials Awareness

cctawareness.org

Advocates for the creation of a federally sponsored public awareness campaign to increase the public's understanding of the benefits of clinical trials.

Colorectal Cancer Alliance

www.ccalliance.org

Provides support for patients and families, caregivers, and survivors; raises awareness of preventive measures; and inspires efforts to fund critical research.

Critical Mass: The Young Adult Cancer Alliance

www.criticalmass.org

Advances policies that will transform the U.S. cancer care and delivery system to better serve adolescent and young adult patients and survivors

Cystic Fibrosis Foundation

www.cff.org

Works to cure cystic fibrosis and to provide all people with the disease the opportunity to lead full, productive lives.

Debbie's Dream Foundation: Curing Stomach Cancer

debbiesdream.org

Dedicated to raising awareness about stomach cancer, advancing funding for research, and providing education and support internationally to patients, families, and caregivers.

Dr. Susan Love Foundation for Breast Cancer Research

drsusanloveresearch.org

Challenges the status quo to end breast cancer and improve the lives of people impacted by it now through education and advocacy.

Family Caregiver Alliance

www.caregiver.org

Works to improve the quality of life for caregivers and those they care for through information, services, and advocacy.

Family Reach

familyreach.org

Alleviates the financial burden of cancer by providing immediate financial assistance, education, and navigation to families before they hit critical breaking points.

Faster Cures

milkeninstitute.org/centers/fastercures

Works to save lives by speeding up and improving the medical research system.

Fight Colorectal Cancer

fightcolorectalcancer.org

Empowers and activates a community of patients, fighters, and champions to push for better policies and to support research, education, and awareness.

FORCE (Facing Our Risk of Cancer Empowered)

www.facingourrisk.org/index.php

Works to improve the lives of individuals and families affected by hereditary cancers.

Global Liver Institute

www.globalliver.org

Improves the lives of individuals and families impacted by liver disease through promoting innovation, encouraging collaboration, and scaling optimal approaches to help eradicate liver diseases.

GO2 Foundation for Lung Cancer

go2foundation.org

Dedicated to saving, extending, and improving the lives of those vulnerable, at risk, and diagnosed with lung cancer.

Head and Neck Cancer Alliance

headandneck.org

Advances prevention, detection, treatment, and rehabilitation of oral, head, and neck cancer through public awareness, research, advocacy, and survivorship.

Imerman Angels

imermanangels.org

Provides comfort and understanding for all cancer fighters, survivors, previvors, and caregivers through a personalized, one on-one connection with someone who has been there.

International Myeloma Foundation (IMF)

www.myeloma.org

Improves the quality of life of myeloma patients while working toward prevention and a cure through four founding principles: research, education, support, and advocacy.

Kidney Cancer Action Network (KidneyCAN)

kidneycan.org

As the voice of kidney cancer advocacy in Washington, DC, and across the United States, KidneyCAN is committed to curing kidney cancer and other cancers now.

Kidney Cancer Association (KCA)

www.kidneycancer.org

A global community dedicated to serving and empowering patients and caregivers, and leading change through advocacy, research, and education.

Kidney Cancer Research Alliance (KCCure)

kccure.org

Dedicated to eliminating suffering and death due to kidney cancer through increased funding to accelerate research that will lead to a cure for all patients and prevent future kidney cancer diagnoses.

Latinas Contra Cancer

latinascontracancer.org,

Provides education, patient navigation, and support for underserved, low-income, and Spanish-speaking women.

LawHelp.org

www.lawhelp.org

Provides assistance in finding legal aid programs to people with low and moderate incomes.

Leukemia and Lymphoma Society (LLS)

www.lls.org

Works to cure leukemia, lymphoma, Hodgkin's disease, and myeloma and improve the quality of life of patients and their families.

Livestrong

www.livestrong.org

Provides direct services, connects people and communities with the services they need, and calls for state, national, and world leaders to help fight cancer.

Living Beyond Breast Cancer (LBBC)

www.lbbc.org

Connects people with trusted breast cancer information and a community of support.

Lung Cancer Research Foundation

www.lungcancerresearchfoundation.org

Improves lung cancer outcomes by funding research for the prevention, diagnosis, treatment, and cure of lung cancer.

LUNGevity

lungevity.org

Committed to increasing quality of life and survivorship of people with lung cancer by accelerating research, as well as providing community, support, and education.

Lymphoma Research Foundation

lymphoma.org

Works to eradicate lymphoma and serve those touched by this disease.

Malecare

malecare.org

Works to improve the lives of people diagnosed with cancer, their families, and communities by making health services safe, available, understandable, and sustainable.

Melanoma International Foundation

melanomainternational.org

Develops personalized strategies with patients so they may live longer, better lives.

Melanoma Research Alliance

www.curemelanoma.org

Accelerates the pace of scientific discovery and its translation in order to eliminate suffering and death due to melanoma.

Melanoma Research Foundation

melanoma.org

Aims to eradicate melanoma by accelerating medical research while educating to and advocating for the melanoma community.

Metastatic Breast Cancer Network (MBCN)

mbcn.org

A volunteer, patient-led advocacy organization that seeks to address the unique needs and concerns of women and men who are living with metastatic or stage IV breast cancer.

METAvivor

www.metavivor.org

Works to transition metastatic breast cancer from a terminal diagnosis to a chronic, manageable disease with a decent quality of life.

Multiple Myeloma Research Foundation (MMRF)

themmrf.org

Fights for a world where every person has precisely what they need to prevent or defeat multiple myeloma whenever they need it.

Musella Foundation

virtualtrials.com/musella.cfm

Dedicated to helping brain tumor patients through emotional and financial support, education, advocacy, and raising money for brain tumor research.

National Alliance for Caregiving (NAC)

www.caregiving.org

Improves quality of life for families and their care recipients through research, innovation, and advocacy.

National Brain Tumor Society (NBTS)

braintumor.org

Committed to finding better treatments, and ultimately a cure, for people living with a brain tumor today and anyone who will be diagnosed tomorrow.

National Breast Cancer Coalition (NBCC)

www.stopbreastcancer.org

Works to end breast cancer through the power of action and advocacy.

National Breast Cancer Foundation

www.nationalbreastcancer.org

Provides early detection screenings, including mammograms; breast health education; and a supportive community.

National Cancer Legal Services Network (NCLSN)

www.nclsn.org

Promotes increased availability of free legal service programs so that people affected by cancer can focus on medical care and their quality of life.

National Cervical Cancer Coalition

www.nccc-online.org

Helps women, family members, and caregivers battle the personal issues related to cervical cancer and HPV, and advocates for cervical health in all women.

National CML Society

www.nationalcmlsociety.org

Brings hope through educational resources, access to chronic myeloid leukemia (CML) specialists, and a living, breathing network of others that can share their personal CML experiences and successes.

National Coalition for Cancer Survivorship (NCCS)

www.canceradvocacy.org

Advocates for quality cancer care for all people touched by cancer.

National LGBT Cancer Network

cancer-network.org

Education, training, and advocacy for LGBT people with cancer and at risk for cancer. Find an LGBT-friendly cancer care facility.

National LGBT Cancer Project

www.lgbtcancer.org

Provides LGBT cancer survivors with peer-to-peer support, patient navigation, education, and advocacy.

National Minority Quality Forum (NMQF)

www.nmqf.org

Assists health care providers, professionals, administrators, researchers, policy makers, and community and faith-based organizations in delivering appropriate health care to minority communities.

National Organization for Rare Diseases (NORD)

rarediseases.org

Committed to the identification, treatment, and cure of rare disorders through programs of education, advocacy, research, and patient services.

National Patient Advocate Foundation (NPAF)

www.npaf.org

Advances person-centered care for everyone facing a serious illness, and advocates for accessible, high-quality, affordable health care.

No Stomach for Cancer

www.nostomachforcancer.org

Supports research and unites the caring power of people worldwide affected by stomach cancer.

Nueva Vida

www.nueva-vida.org

Informs, supports, and empowers Latinas whose lives are affected by cancer, and advocates for and facilitates the timely access to state-of-the-art cancer care.

Ovarian Cancer Research Alliance

ocrahope.org

Advances ovarian cancer research while supporting women and their families.

Pancreatic Cancer Action Network (PanCAN)

www.pancan.org

Attacks pancreatic cancer on all fronts: research, clinical initiatives, patient services, and advocacy.

Patient Access Network Foundation (PAN)

www.panfoundation.org

Helps underinsured people with life-threatening, chronic, and rare diseases get the medications and treatment they need by paying for their out-of-pocket costs and advocating for improved access and affordability.

Patient Advocate Foundation (PAF)

www.patientadvocate.org

Seeks to safeguard patients through effective mediation, assuring access to care, maintenance of employment, and preservation of their financial stability.

Prevent Cancer Foundation

www.preventcancer.org

Saves lives across all populations through cancer prevention and early detection.

Prostate Cancer Foundation

www.pcf.org

Funds the world's most promising research to improve the prevention, detection, and treatment of prostate cancer and ultimately cure it for good.

Prostate Cancer Research Institute

pcri.org

Improves the quality of prostate cancer patients' and caregivers' lives by empowering them to manage their prostate cancer through education.

Research Advocacy Network (RAN)

researchadvocacy.org

Advances patient-focused cancer research by fostering interaction among advocates, researchers, and related organizations.

Rosalynn Carter Institute for Caregiving

www.rosalynncarter.org

Committed to building quality, long-term, home- and community-based services by providing caregivers with effective supports to promote caregiver health, skills, and resilience.

SHARE Cancer Support

www.sharecancersupport.org

Creates and sustains a supportive network and community of women affected by breast and ovarian cancers.

Sisters Network

www.sistersnetworkinc.org

Committed to increasing local and national attention to the devastating impact that breast cancer has in the African American community.

Skin Cancer Foundation

www.skincancer.org

Empowers people to take a proactive approach to daily sun protection and early detection and treatment of skin cancer.

Stupid Cancer

stupidcancer.org

Empowers, supports, and improves health outcomes for the young adult cancer community.

Support for People with Oral and Head and Neck Cancer (SPOHNC)

www.spohnc.org

Dedicated to raising awareness and meeting the needs of oral and head and neck cancer patients through its resources and publications.

Susan G. Komen Breast Cancer Foundation

ww5.komen.org

Saves lives by meeting the most critical needs in our communities and investing in breakthrough research to prevent and cure breast cancer.

Testicular Cancer Foundation

testicularcancer.org

Provides education and support to young adult males to raise awareness about testicular cancer.

ThyCa: Thyroid Cancer Survivors' Association

www.thyca.org

Dedicated to support, education, and communication for thyroid cancer survivors, their families, and friends.

Triage Cancer

triagecancer.org

Works to address cancer-related health disparities through the delivery of cancer survivorship education, particularly information related to accessing care.

Ulman Foundation

ulmanfoundation.org

Changes lives by creating a community of support for young adults, and their loved ones, impacted by cancer.

Urology Care Foundation

www.urologyhealth.org

Supports urologic research and strives to provide the most current, comprehensive, and reliable urologic health information for patients and the public.

UsTOO International

www.ustoo.org/Home

Provides hope and improves the lives of those affected by prostate cancer through support, education, and advocacy/awareness.

Young Survival Coalition (YSC)

www.youngsurvival.org

Dedicated to the critical issues unique to young women who are diagnosed with breast cancer. YSC offers resources, connections, and outreach so women feel supported, empowered, and hopeful.

Zero: The End of Prostate Cancer

zerocancer.org

Advances research, improves the lives of men and families, and inspires action to end prostate cancer

FEDERAL AND STATE PROGRAMS: INSURANCE AND EMPLOYMENT

Medicare
www.medicare.gov
800-Medicare
Get information about Medicare coverage, eligibility, and costs and plan finders for supplemental/gap and Part D plans.

Social Security Administration
www.ssa.gov
800-772-1213
Apply for Social Security Disability Income (SSDI) or Supplemental Security Income (SSI), as well as Medicare savings programs for qualified beneficiaries and the Extra Help Program for Part D prescription assistance.

State Disability Programs
Five states (California, Hawaii, New Jersey, New York, Rhode Island) and Puerto Rico offer state disability insurance to replace income for workers who are unable to work due to illness. Guidelines vary from state to state. For more information, contact state agencies:

- **California:** disability leave: 800-480-3287; paid family leave: 877-238-4373
- **Hawaii:** 808-586-9161
- **New Jersey:** 609-292-7060

- **New York:** 800-353-3092
- **Puerto Rico:** 787-754-2142
- **Rhode Island:** 401-462-8420

COBRA

www.dol.gov/agencies/ebsa/laws-and-regulations/laws/cobra
866-4-USA-DOL
COBRA contains provisions giving certain former employees, retirees, spouses, former spouses, and dependent children the right to temporary continuation of health coverage at group rates. This coverage, however, is available only when coverage is lost due to certain specific events; overseen by the Department of Labor.

Family and Medical Leave Act (FMLA)

www.dol.gov/agencies/whd/fmla
The Family and Medical Leave Act (FMLA) provides job protections for time away from work due to illness or caregiving needs. Federal law applies to employers with fifty or more employees. Some states have different guidelines. Talk directly to your employer about your FMLA options. For general FMLA information, see the website above.

State Health Insurance Assistance Programs (SHIPS)

www.shiptacenter.org/about-us/about-ships
State Health Insurance Assistance Programs (SHIPs) provide free, in-depth, one-on-one insurance counseling and assistance to Medicare beneficiaries, their families, friends, and caregivers.

Children's Health Insurance Program (CHIP)

www.medicaid.gov/chip/index.html
The Children's Health Insurance Program (CHIP) provides health coverage to eligible children, through both Medicaid and separate CHIP programs. CHIP is administered by states, according to federal requirements. The program is funded jointly by states and the federal government.

Veterans

www.va.gov/healthbenefits
Eligible veterans may be able to receive health care coverage through the Veterans Administration.

Medicaid

www.medicaid.gov/medicaid/index.html

Medicaid provides health coverage to millions of Americans, including eligible low-income adults, children, pregnant women, elderly adults, and people with disabilities. Medicaid is administered by states, according to federal requirements. The program is funded jointly by states and the federal government.

Affordable Care Act / Healthcare Marketplace

www.healthcare.gov

The Affordable Care Act ("Obamacare") / Healthcare Marketplace offers health insurance options for those who do not qualify for Medicaid, Medicare, veterans' benefits, or employer-affiliated health insurance plans.

Equal Employment Opportunity Commission

www.eeoc.gov

800-669-4000

Investigates workplace discrimination claims.

Job Accommodation Network

askjan.org

Assists with workplace accommodations and navigation of the Americans with Disabilities Act (ADA).

RESOURCES FOR FINANCIAL SUPPORT

FINANCIAL ASSISTANCE

There are many different local and national resources for financial assistance, but the programs are always changing. To get help finding ones that might be helpful to you, contact the Cancer Support Community Helpline at 888-793-9355.

National Co-pay and Financial Assistance from Nonprofit Organizations

Some nonprofit organizations provide funding for co-pays only for people who are underinsured. They generally do not provide help paying for treatment to individuals who are uninsured. Many nonprofits also provide funding for other out-of-pocket costs, such as insurance premiums, transportation, lodging, home care, childcare, diagnosis, and even pet assistance. Diseases covered and services offered vary among organizations. There may also be financial aid available in your area for utilities, rent, or other living costs. To get help finding what resources might be available for you, contact the Cancer Support Community Helpline at 888-793-9355.

The Assistance Fund
tafcares.org
855-845-3663
Financial assistance for medication costs, co-pays, insurance premiums, and travel expenses.

CancerCare Co-payment Assistance Foundation
www.cancercare.org/copayfoundation
866-55-COPAY
Financial assistance for treatment and prescription co-pays.

CancerCare Financial Assistance Program
www.cancercare.org/financial
800-813-4673
Limited financial assistance for cancer-related costs such as transportation, childcare, home care, and pet costs.

Good Days
www.mygooddays.org
(877) 968-7233
Financial assistance for co-pays, insurance premiums, diagnostic costs, and travel expenses.

HealthWell Foundation
www.healthwellfoundation.org
800-675-8416
Financial assistance for co-pays, prescriptions, insurance premiums, and travel expenses.

Leukemia and Lymphoma Society Financial Support
www.lls.org/support/financial-support
800-955-4572
Financial assistance for insurance premiums, treatment co-pays, and prescription costs. Small financial aid grants and travel assistance.

National Association for Rare Disorders (NORD)
rarediseases.org
800-999-6673
Financial assistance for medication, insurance premiums, co-pays, diagnostic testing, and travel expenses.

Patient Access Network Foundation (PAN)

www.panfoundation.org

866-316-7263

Financial assistance for medication costs, co-pays, insurance premiums, and travel expenses.

Patient Advocate Foundation Co-Pay Relief

copays.org

866-512-3861

Financial assistance for co-pays.

Patient Advocate Foundation Financial Aid Funds

www.patientadvocate.org/connect-with-services/financial-aid-funds

800-532-5274

Small, onetime financial aid grants.

Patient Services Incorporated

www.patientservicesinc.org

800-366-7741

Financial assistance for insurance premiums, co-pays, and travel expenses.

PHARMACEUTICAL MANUFACTURER ASSISTANCE

There are different types of assistance available through many pharmaceutical companies:

- For individuals with some prescription coverage who still have problems affording their share of drug costs, co-pay assistance or discount cards may be available from each company that makes the drugs you are receiving.
- For individuals with little or no insurance coverage of their cancer drug costs, patient assistance may be available from the drug company. You or your health care team will need to contact the drug company directly for its guidelines and application.

To get help finding the most up-to-date information on drug company assistance programs, contact the Cancer Support Community Helpline at 888-793-9355.

The Association of Community Cancer Centers (ACCC) keeps an up-to-date, comprehensive list of cancer drug patient assistance programs by the name of the drug company on its website: www.accc-cancer.org/home/learn/publications/patient -assistance-and-reimbursement-guide.

GLOSSARY

Also refer to the NCI Dictionary of Cancer Terms at www.cancer.gov/publications/dictionaries/cancer-terms.

ablation: The removal or destruction of a body part or tissue or its function.

active surveillance: A treatment plan that involves closely watching a patient's condition but not giving any treatment unless there are changes in test results that show the condition is getting worse. Active surveillance may be used to avoid or delay the need for treatments such as radiation therapy or surgery, which can cause side effects or other problems. During active surveillance, certain exams and tests are done on a regular schedule. Also called watch and wait.

acupuncture: The technique of inserting thin needles through the skin at specific points on the body to control pain and other symptoms. It is a type of complementary and alternative medicine.

adjuvant therapy: Treatment given after the first or primary treatment (which is often surgery).

adjuvant trials: Research studies done after primary treatment for cancer (such as surgery or radiation therapy) to reduce the chance the cancer will recur or come back.

advance directive: A legal document containing written instructions about a person's future medical care if they become unable to express their wishes.

adverse event (AE): Any unfavorable change in a patient's health while on treatment. This includes abnormal lab findings, side effects of the treatment, and health problems that may not be caused by the treatment but happen during or after a person receives that treatment.

advocate: A person who provides support and information to, in this case, people with cancer. Advocates participate in the cancer community in many different ways.

allogeneic or "allo" stem cell transplant: A stem cell transplant using the healthy stem cells from a family member or matching donor. (Also see *stem cell transplant*.)

alopecia: Hair loss during cancer treatment that is almost always temporary and grows back when therapy is finished.

alternative therapy: Nontraditional methods of diagnosing, preventing, or treating cancer that are used instead of proven methods.

Americans with Disabilities Act (ADA): A federal law that prohibits discrimination against people with disabilities. It requires employers to make "reasonable accommodations" (see definition) in the workplace for individuals deemed to have a disability. "Disability," for purposes of the ADA, means that a person has, has a history of, or is regarded as having a physical or mental impairment that substantially limits one or more major life activities that the average person in the general population can perform. The ADA doesn't include a list of conditions that are "disabilities." It is determined on an individual basis.

anemia: A shortage of red blood cells that can cause weakness and fatigue.

angiogenesis: Blood vessel formation. Tumor angiogenesis is the growth of blood vessels from surrounding tissue to a solid tumor. This is caused by the release of chemicals by the tumor.

angiogenesis inhibitor therapy: Treatment to prevent development of new blood vessels that supply blood to the tumor, thereby stopping or limiting tumor growth.

annual (insurance) limit: The amount an insurance plan will pay in total benefits over one plan year. Once a patient's medical bills reach the total or "cap" for the year, the policy will not pay again until the following year. Sometimes there are annual caps for particular services such as home health. The Affordable Care Act (ACA) now prohibits annual limits on essential health benefits for all plans except grandfathered individual plans.

antibody: A protein made by the body's immune cells to attach to a specific foreign invader, such as bacteria, viruses, and potentially cancerous cells.

appeal: A method of disputing the denial of a claim made to an insurance plan for payment of a service. A patient can appeal any claim denied by their medical insurance provider. This process may vary according to the insurance plan.

arm: A group of participants in a study who are receiving the same treatment.

autologous or "auto" stem cell transplant: A stem cell transplant using a patient's own stem cells. (Also see *stem cell transplant*.)

benign: Not cancer.

biomarker: A substance in blood, bodily fluid, or cells that doctors measure to learn more about a person's cancer.

biomarker testing: Testing that looks for changes in a cancer's genes. It helps doctors match targeted therapies to the specific subtype of cancer. A sample of the cancer is collected via bodily fluids, surgery, or biopsy and sent to a lab. Test results can then be used to help guide treatment options. For example, biomarker test results will show if a patient is *ALK+* in lung cancer, *HER2+* in breast cancer, or *BRAF+* in melanoma or colorectal cancer. Also called tumor profiling, genomic testing, mutation testing, or molecular testing.

biopsy: The removal of cells or tissues for examination by a pathologist to see whether cancer is present. The pathologist may study the tissue under a microscope or perform other tests on the cells or tissue.

blinding: Setting up a clinical trial so that neither the doctors nor the participants know who is getting which treatment.

bone scan: A method of imaging using a radioactive tracer that looks for cancer or other changes in the bone.

brachytherapy: A type of radiation therapy in which radioactive material sealed in needles, seeds, wires, or catheters is placed directly into or near a tumor. Also called implant radiation therapy, internal radiation therapy, or radiation brachytherapy.

brand-name medication: Prescription medications are usually initially marketed under a specific brand name by the company that holds the patent. When patents run out, generic versions of many medications are marketed at lower cost by other companies.

bronchoscopy: A bronchoscope (a flexible tubelike instrument) is used to directly view the airways into the lungs and to collect tissue samples. Local anesthesia and mild sedation are generally used.

cancer subtype: Describes the smaller groups that a type of cancer can be divided into, based on certain characteristics of the cancer cells. These characteristics include how the cancer cells look under a microscope and whether there are certain substances in or on the cells or certain changes to the DNA of the cells. It is important to know the subtype of a cancer to plan treatment and determine prognosis.

cancer type: Cancer is generally named by the organ or cell where it starts. Lung cancer and breast cancer are cancer types.

chemo brain: Common term used to describe thinking and memory problems experienced during and after cancer treatments.

chemotherapy: Treatment with drugs to stop the growth of rapidly dividing cancer cells.

chemotherapy cycle: Term used to describe the process in which chemotherapy is given, followed by a period of rest in which the body is allowed to recover.

chemotherapy regimen: Combinations of anticancer drugs given at a certain dose in a specific order according to a strict schedule.

chest X-ray: An X-ray of the structures inside the chest. An X-ray is a type of high-energy radiation that can go through the body and onto film, making pictures of areas inside the chest, which can be used to diagnose disease.

clinical trial or clinical study: A research study to test how well new medical treatments work in people. Each clinical trial tests new ways of screening, preventing, diagnosing, or treating cancer, or improving quality of life for people with cancer.

clinical trial, phase I (1): The first test of the dose and safety of a drug. Doctors work with small groups of patients who may have different kinds of cancer. Many phase I trials are for people with cancers that have spread to other parts of their bodies.

clinical trial, phase II (2): Phase II trials are done if a phase I trial showed that the treatment is safe and works against one or more types of cancer. A phase II trial is a larger study, often done with specific cancer types. It looks at how well a treatment can work in that type of cancer.

clinical trial, phase III (3): Phase III trials are large studies. They involve hundreds of thousands of patients. These studies are often done in many cancer centers in the United States or around the world. For this phase, patients are assigned to get either the new treatment or the "standard of care" (current base treatment). In order to give everyone an equal chance at the new treatment, a computer decides randomly which treatment each patient will get. The doctor does not have any role in deciding which patients get which treatments and often does not know who is getting the standard of care.

clinical trial, phase IV (4): Phase IV trials occur after a drug or new treatment is approved. Doctors continue to monitor it to learn how it works over the long term. They also look to see if there are any side effects that appear months or even years after treatment.

COBRA: The Consolidated Omnibus Budget Reconciliation Act (COBRA) is a federal law that allows individuals who lose their jobs or experience another qualifying event to keep their health insurance coverage for an extended period of time, if they meet certain criteria and pay the premiums.

coinsurance: The percentage of costs an insured patient pays after meeting a health care plan's annual deductible. For example, an 80/20 coinsurance rate means that the insurance company pays 80 percent of approved health care costs and the patient pays out of pocket the remaining 20 percent of costs. Coinsurance usually does not start until the insured pays an amount equal to a deductible.

colorectal: Having to do with the colon and/or rectum.

combination therapy: The use of more than one form of treatment at the same time.

complete blood count (CBC): The complete blood count (CBC) test counts the number and types of blood cells in a sample of blood.

complete response (CR): The removal of all signs of cancer in response to treatment. This does not necessarily mean that a patient is cured.

controlled trial: A study in which the new treatment is compared to a control (usually the standard of care).

co-payment (co-pay): A dollar amount set by an insurance provider that a patient is required to pay each time care is received. For example, a visit to the doctor may cost a patient thirty dollars each time, and the insurance company will pay the balance of the visit's cost. The amount of the co-pay is set by the insurance provider and not the doctor's office.

cryoablation: A process in which liquid nitrogen or argon gas is used to freeze tumors.

CT scan (CAT scan): A series of detailed pictures of areas inside the body, taken from different angles. The pictures are created by a computer linked to an X-ray machine.

deductible: The amount of approved health care costs an insured patient must pay out of pocket each year before the health care plan begins paying any costs.

dermatology: The branch of medicine focused on the skin.

disease progression: Term used to describe the growth or spread of cancer.

disease-free survival: The time from when a person with no detectable cancer begins a treatment until the cancer appears or returns.

do-not-resuscitate (DNR) order: An instruction in a patient's chart, written by their doctor, that tells other doctors and medical staff that the patient would not like CPR if their heart stops or if they stop breathing.

donut hole: A commonly used term for the coverage gap in the Medicare Part D prescription drug benefit.

driver mutations: Changes in a cancer cell's genes that cause or "drive" the cancer to grow, divide, and spread. Some causes of these changes are known (e.g., tobacco use, harmful chemicals, aging), but others are not.

durable power of attorney: A person who can make health care decisions for a patient if they can't make them on their own.

dysphagia: Difficulty swallowing.

dyspnea: Difficult, painful breathing, or shortness of breath.

eligibility requirements: Every clinical trial has certain standards that people must meet in order to participate. These usually are related to the kind and stage of cancer, any previous treatments, and overall health.

endocrinology: The branch of medicine focused on the endocrine glands and hormones.

esophagitis: Condition caused by radiation treatment that results in the symptoms of painful and difficult swallowing. Often described as a feeling of food getting stuck in the throat.

exclusion criteria: Factors that can make a person not eligible or able to participate in a clinical trial.

explanation of benefits (EOB): A document from an insurance administrator that outlines what portion of the provider's charges are eligible for benefits under an insurance plan. An EOB is not a bill, but it explains what was covered by insurance. A provider may bill the patient separately for any charges the person is still responsible for.

fatigue: Decreased capacity for activity that is often accompanied by feelings of weariness, sleepiness, or irritability.

federally insured plan: See *HIPAA plan*.

first-line therapy: The initial cancer treatment. Second-line therapy may follow if the first line is not successful or stops working, and so on.

Food and Drug Administration (FDA): The federal agency responsible for assuring that all drugs and medical devices available in the United States are safe and effective. The FDA reviews—but does not conduct—clinical trials.

formulary: A list of prescription medications that an insurance company prefers to cover. Health insurance company formularies usually include most generic medications but only a selection of brand-name drugs. "On formulary" refers to drugs covered by a specific insurance company.

free clinic: According to the National Association of Free Clinics, "Free clinics are volunteer-based, safety-net health care organizations that provide a range of medical, dental, pharmacy, and/or behavioral health services to economically disadvantaged individuals who are predominately uninsured. Free clinics are 501(c)(3) tax-exempt organizations, or operate as a program component or affiliate of a 501(c)(3) organization. Entities that otherwise meet the above definition, but charge a nominal fee to patients, may still be considered free clinics provided essential services are delivered regardless of the patient's ability to pay."

gastroenterology: The branch of medicine focused on the gastrointestinal tract (stomach, intestines, etc.) and liver.

gene: Pieces of DNA present in every cell in the body.

generic medication: Once the patent on a brand-name medication has run out, other drug companies are allowed to sell a version of the drug that is a duplicate of the original. Generic drugs are typically cheaper, and most prescription and health plans encourage use of generics.

genetic marker: A gene or piece of DNA associated with a certain disease.

genetic testing for inheritable cancer risk: The process of analyzing the genes and chromosomes inherited from a person's parents to see if changes (mutations) are a sign that the person has an increased risk of developing cancer.

genomic testing: See *biomarker testing*.

grade: In cancer, a description of a tumor based on how abnormal the cancer cells and tissue look under a microscope and how quickly the cancer cells are likely to grow and spread. Low-grade cancer cells look more like normal cells and tend to grow and spread more slowly than high-grade cancer cells. Grading systems are different for each type of cancer. They are used to help plan treatment and determine prognosis. Also called histologic grade and tumor grade.

group policy: Group insurance is usually offered through an employer or some form of a trade association. It provides certain benefits that individual policies do not.

G-tube: A tube inserted through the wall of the abdomen into the stomach. It can be used to give drugs and liquids, including liquid food.

guaranteed issue plan: A health insurance policy issued regardless of a person's age, gender, income, or medical conditions.

gynecology: The branch of medicine focused on the female reproductive organs.

hematology: The branch of medicine focused on blood.

HIPAA plan: A law that protects patient privacy.

histology: Study of tissues to determine their specific characteristics, which may lead to identifying a specific subtype of cancer.

home health care: Health care provided by a skilled professional such as a nurse, social worker, or physical therapist in a home setting.

hormone therapy: Treatment that adds, blocks, or removes hormones. For certain conditions (such as diabetes or menopause), hormones are given to adjust low hormone levels. Hormones can also cause certain cancers (such as prostate and breast cancer) to grow. To slow or stop the growth of cancer, synthetic hormones or other drugs may be given to block the body's natural hormones, or surgery may be used to remove the gland that makes a certain hormone. Also called endocrine therapy, hormone therapy, or hormone treatment.

hospice: End-of-life care given after treatment has been ended; focuses on making the patient and family members feel comfortable and supported.

human subjects review board: See *institutional review board (IRB)*.

immune system: A network of cells, tissues, and organs that work together to protect the body from bacteria, viruses, parasites, fungi, and abnormal cells like cancer.

immunotherapy: Cancer treatment that works by boosting the body's natural immune response.

inclusion criteria: The factors that allow a person to participate in a study.

informed consent: The formal process researchers use to make sure patients understand a clinical trial and fully agree to participate in it. This is an important way of communicating with patients and caregivers about the goals of the study, possible results, and side effects. The process also provides an opportunity to ask questions.

in-network: See *preferred providers*.

institutional review board (IRB): The group at a medical center that reviews all proposed clinical trials taking place in that center to make sure they are safe and effective for patients and that all patients' rights are protected.

investigational new drug: A drug or agent that is being used in a clinical trial but has not yet been approved by the FDA.

investigator: A researcher who is conducting a clinical trial.

liquid biopsy: A new technology that allows the detection of tumor DNA in the blood for biomarker analysis. It doesn't identify stage, is currently not as sensitive as other types of biopsies, and is best not used alone (without other types of biopsy).

living will: A legal document that details a person's wishes about medical treatment if a time should come when they can no longer express those wishes.

locally advanced: Describes a cancer that has spread to nearby tissue or lymph nodes but not outside the local area where the cancer started.

lymph nodes: Glands found all over the body that help fight infection. Cancer often spreads to lymph nodes.

lymphedema: A side effect of some cancer treatment that causes swelling in the lymph nodes, often in the arms or legs.

maintenance therapy: Lower-intensity therapy given after first-line therapy to delay the return of cancer.

malignant: Cancerous. Malignant cells can invade and destroy nearby tissue and spread to other parts of the body.

Medicaid: A government-funded health insurance available to individuals and families who can demonstrate need as established through income and asset standards. The program is jointly funded by states and the federal government and administered by states. Medicaid eligibility and benefits vary from state to state.

medical power of attorney: Document that allows an individual to appoint a trusted person to make decisions about their medical care if they cannot make decisions on their own.

Medicare: A government-funded health insurance usually available to U.S. citizens sixty-five years of age and over and those who have been receiving Social Security disability benefits for twenty-four months. Medicare benefits are the same, regardless of where a person lives in the United States.

Medigap: A Medigap policy is health insurance sold by private insurance companies to fill the "gaps" in Original Medicare plan coverage. Medigap policies help pay some of the health care costs that Original Medicare doesn't cover.

metastasis: The spread of cancer to other tissues.

metastatic: Having to do with metastasis, the spread of cancer from its original location to another part of the body.

metastatic cancer: Stage IV or advanced cancer. Cancer that has spread from its original location to another, distant part of the body.

minimum essential coverage: The type of health insurance coverage a person needs to have in order to meet the Affordable Care Act (ACA) law that requires most U.S. citizens and those lawfully present in the United States to have health insurance coverage. Minimum essential coverage includes individual policies, employer-sponsored policies, Medicare, Medicaid, CHIP, TRICARE, and certain other types of coverage.

molecular marker: Another term for biomarker (see definition).

molecular testing: See *biomarker testing*.

monoclonal antibodies: Substances produced in a laboratory and tailored to attach themselves to a specific protein (antigen), attacking and destroying only tumor cells.

MRI (magnetic resonance imaging): A procedure in which radio waves and a powerful magnet linked to a computer are used to create detailed pictures of areas inside the body. These pictures can show the difference between normal and diseased tissue. Also called nuclear magnetic resonance imaging (NMRI).

multimodality or combined modality therapy: Treatment using a combination of chemotherapy, surgery, radiation therapy, immunotherapy, and/or targeted therapy.

mutation: A change in a cell's genes (DNA).

mutation testing: See *biomarker testing*.

navigational bronchoscopy: This new technology uses a bronchoscope to provide a three-dimensional virtual "road map" that enables a doctor to biopsy hard-to-reach parts of the lungs.

needle biopsy: A procedure in which a small piece of tissue is removed and viewed under a microscope. This may be taken from the lung or a part of the body where the cancer has spread.

neoadjuvant therapy: Chemotherapy or radiation therapy used before surgery to shrink a tumor.

neoadjuvant trials: Clinical trials done to test treatments (like chemotherapy) before the primary treatment for a cancer (such as surgery or radiation therapy). This is done to eliminate or reduce the amount of cancer.

nephrology: The branch of medicine focused on the kidneys.

neurology: The branch of medicine focused on the central nervous system (brain, spinal cord, and nerves).

neuropathy: A condition marked by sometimes severe discomfort in the nerves that can be a symptom of cancer or side effect of cancer treatment.

no evidence of disease (NED): A patient's status when there are no longer any visual signs of cancer on diagnostic tests like CT scans or PET Scans. This does not mean that all the cancer is gone from the body. It just means that the cancer may be too small to see with the current methods of imaging.

off-label: The use of a medication for a purpose other than the use approved by the U.S. Food and Drug Administration (FDA). The FDA approves drugs as safe and effective for specific uses—for example, use for colon cancer or breast cancer. More than half of the uses of anticancer medications are for indications that are not specified as approved or indicated on the label. Some insurance companies may deny coverage for a medication that is used off-label. The federal government requires that Medicare cover these off-label uses for treating life-threatening conditions as long as certain requirements are met. This is true for many private insurers as well.

oncology: The branch of medicine focused on cancer and tumors.

open biopsy: A surgical procedure in which a tissue sample is taken.

open enrollment: Open enrollment is a period of time, usually occurring once per year, when employees of U.S. companies and organizations may make additions, changes, or deletions to their health insurance coverage and other benefits. In most cases, employees can make changes in benefits elections only during open enrollment or when they have experienced a specific qualifying event. Medicare and the state health insurance marketplaces also have open enrollment periods.

ophthalmology: The branch of medicine focused on the eye.

osteoporosis: A condition that is characterized by a decrease in bone mass and density, causing bones to become fragile. Some cancer treatments put women at higher risk for developing osteoporosis.

out-of-pocket expenses: The portion of health care expenses a patient must pay when a treatment or service is not covered by insurance. This may include expenses directly related to treatment such as doctor visits, laboratory tests, X-rays, and medications, as well as those that may not be directly related to medical care, such as transportation to the doctor's office or hospital, parking, or childcare.

overall survival: The length of time a person lives from the beginning of treatment.

oxygen therapy: A treatment used to relieve breathing problems by providing supplemental oxygen.

palliative care: A medical specialty that focuses on symptom management and quality of life.

palliative therapy: A treatment used to relieve pain and other symptoms without the intent to cure the disease.

partial remission: The status of a cancer that has responded to treatment but not totally disappeared. The cancer can still be detected, and other treatments may be recommended.

partial response: The reduction in the size of a cancer tumor by at least 50 percent.

pathologic complete response (pCR): The total disappearance of a cancer following neoadjuvant therapy. This is an important way for researchers to measure the outcomes of a neoadjuvant clinical trial.

pathologist: A doctor who specializes in diagnosing specific diseases by examining cells and tissues under a microscope.

pathology: The branch of medicine focused on laboratory examination of samples of body tissue.

pathology report: A medical report that gives information about a diagnosis. To test for cancer, a sample of tissue is sent to a lab. There, a doctor called a pathologist studies it under a microscope and may do tests to get more information.

peripheral neuropathy: Damage to the nervous system. Some chemotherapy drugs can cause this condition. Symptoms include weakness or tingling in the hands or feet.

PET (positron emission tomography) scan: A procedure in which a small amount of radioactive glucose (sugar) is injected into a vein and a scanner is used to make detailed computerized pictures of areas inside the body where the glucose is taken up. Because cancer cells often take up more glucose than normal cells, the pictures can be used to find cancer cells in the body.

placebo: An inactive substance, sometimes called a "sugar pill." Placebos are almost never used in cancer clinical trials. Most studies involve getting the standard of care for the specific cancer type.

pleural effusion: Abnormal collection of fluid between the thin layers of tissue (pleura) lining the lung and the wall of the chest cavity.

power of attorney: A legal document that authorizes a person to make legal and financial decisions on behalf of another person.

pre-authorization: Managed care–type health insurance policies may require a patient to request approval from the plan for specific services before the services are provided. This may include a treatment, procedure, or hospital stay. Case managers may be able to help with this process.

precision medicine: A process to find the best treatments for each specific patient based on exact gene changes or proteins in their cancer. Doctors test for biomarkers, cell changes (mutations), or other targets found in or on a patient's cancer cells. Then treatments are offered that target the specific biomarker or mutation found in the cancer. These "targeted" drugs are expected to work better. Sometimes called personalized medicine.

preclinical studies: Research done on new drugs and treatments before they are used in humans.

preexisting condition: A medical condition that a person has prior to being covered by new insurance. Health insurance companies and health plans are no longer able to deny coverage based on a person's preexisting condition or impose a preexisting condition exclusion period.

preferred drug list: See *formulary*.

preferred provider: A doctor or hospital that is part of a network of providers approved by a health insurance plan. If a person is enrolled in a preferred provider organization (PPO) or a point-of-service (POS) plan, their out-of-pocket expenses will be less if they use a provider who is part of the plan. They will still get some reimbursement if they receive a covered service from a provider who is not in the network.

premium: The amount a person or company pays each month to maintain insurance coverage.

preventive services: Medical services provided to prevent or detect illness, such as mammograms. Under the Affordable Care Act (ACA), eligible individuals no longer have to pay co-pays, meet their deductibles, or pay coinsurance amounts for specific preventive services. A list is available at HealthCare.gov.

primary care provider (PCP): The doctor a person would normally see first when a health problem comes up. A primary care doctor could be a general practitioner, a family practice doctor, a gynecologist, a pediatrician, or an internal medicine doctor.

primary site or primary cancer: The part of the body where the cancer starts.

primary therapy: The first therapy given after a diagnosis of cancer.

prognosis: The likely outcome of a disease, including the chance of recovery.

progression-free survival: The time from when a patient begins taking a treatment until the cancer begins to grow or spread again.

progressive disease: Disease in which the tumor is growing in spite of the treatment received. When this happens, that specific therapy is usually stopped or modified in some way.

protocol: The written plan or design for a trial that tells doctors what treatments and doses patients get on a study. It is the doctor's recipe for conducting the trial.

psychotherapy: Treatment of mental, emotional, personality, and behavioral issues and disorders using methods such as discussion, listening, and counseling. Also called talk therapy.

pulmonology: The branch of medicine focused on the lungs.

qualifying event: With respect to COBRA eligibility, the event, such as leaving a job or divorce, that makes a person eligible for COBRA coverage. The length of available COBRA coverage depends on the qualifying event.

quality of life: A way of measuring treatments and the patient experience that focuses on a patient's overall health, ability to live and enjoy life, and sense of well-being.

radiation therapy: A procedure in which high doses of high-energy radiation beams (X-rays) are carefully focused on a tumor to kill cancer cells.

randomized: Describes clinical trials in which a computer randomly assigns participants to treatment groups to determine who will get which treatment. Many trials are randomized to make sure that there is no bias in the study. This assures that every patient has an equal chance of getting either the standard of care or the new treatment being tested.

reasonable accommodations: The reasonable efforts that, under the Americans with Disabilities Act (ADA), an employer must make to allow an employee who has been determined to be disabled to continue working. What is "reasonable" depends on the specifics of each situation.

recurrence: The return of a previous cancer.

referral: A doctor's recommendation that a patient see another doctor, usually a specialist.

refractory: Describes a cancer that does not respond to treatment.

relapse: The return of cancer after it has been treated and the person has been in remission.

remission: Absence of disease. A person is in remission when the cancer has been treated and tumors have diminished by at least 50 percent (partial) or have disappeared (complete). Remission does not necessarily mean the disease has been cured.

signature molecule: Another term for biomarker (see definition).

single-agent trials: Studies that test one drug.

specialty pharmacy: A pharmacy that offers additional services and resources, often related to cancer or other chronic illnesses.

sputum cytology: A test in which a sample of sputum (mucus produced by a cough) is collected and looked at under a microscope.

stable disease: Cancer that does not get better or worse following therapy.

stage: The extent of cancer in the body, including whether the disease has spread from the original site to other body sites.

standard of care: Treatment that is widely accepted and used by medical professionals as the treatment for a disease. It is understood as the "best available care."

standard therapy: See *standard of care*.

stem cell transplant: A nonsurgical procedure in which a patient receives an infusion of blood-forming cells (stem cells). A stem cell transplant allows a health care team to use higher-dose chemotherapy than would otherwise be safe to give. The process starts by collecting and freezing healthy blood-forming cells (stem cells) from the patient or a donor. A few rounds of high-dose chemotherapy are then used to kill cancer cells in the body. After this, the stem cells collected earlier are infused into the patient to replace the blood-forming cells that are killed off by the high-dose chemotherapy.

step therapy: The practice of first prescribing the most cost-effective and safest drug therapy for a medical condition. Only if the initially prescribed medication does not work does the patient progress to other, more costly or risky, therapies. The aims are to control costs and minimize risks.

stereotactic radiosurgery: The use of high-energy X-rays to destroy cancer.

stoma: A surgically created opening from an area inside the body to the outside. In head and neck cancer, people who have had their larynx removed breathe through a stoma in their neck. In bladder cancer, people who have had their bladder removed may pass their urine through a stoma in their abdomen. In colorectal cancer, people who have had intestinal surgery may eliminate stool through a stoma in the abdomen.

subtype: See *cancer subtype*.

systemic therapy: Treatments that travel through the bloodstream to reach the whole body, not just a specific organ or body part.

T cell: A type of white blood cell. T cells are the immune system's "soldiers." They help protect the body from infection and can help fight cancer. Also called T lymphocyte.

targeted therapies: Drugs that target specific cellular pathways that enable cancer cells to grow.

thoracentesis: A procedure in which a doctor relieves fluid buildup around the lungs (called pleural effusion) by using a needle to remove some of the fluid. This can help a patient breathe better by expanding the lungs. A sample of the fluid can be sent to a lab to be tested for cancer cells.

thoracic: Related to the part of the body between the neck and abdomen.

tiered: In prescription medication insurance policies, the varying levels of coverage.

TNM staging system: Three measures of tumor spread and size, lymph nodes affected, and metastatic (distant) sites involved that are used to stage cancers at levels I through IV (1 through 4).

toxicity: Harmful side effects that result from an agent being tested.

tumor: An abnormal mass or swelling of tissue. A tumor may occur anywhere in the body. It may be benign (harmless) or malignant (cancerous).

tumor antigen: A substance produced by a tumor cell that can cause the body to create a specific immune response.

tumor marker: A measurable sign (often a protein) in the blood or bodily fluid that may indicate the presence of cancer. It may be used to tell if a treatment is working. Examples of tumor markers include CA 15-3 (breast cancer) and CEA (ovarian, lung, breast, pancreas, and gastrointestinal tract cancers).

tumor profiling: See *biomarker testing*.

urology: The branch of medicine focused on the male and female urinary tract and male reproductive tract.

usual and customary: The typical or average cost for health care services within a specific geographic area. Usual and customary is often used by an insurance plan to decide how much it will pay for specific services. If a doctor's charges for services are higher than this average, the patient may have to pay the difference.

vascular endothelial growth factor (VEGF): A protein that stimulates new blood vessel formation. VEGF inhibitors block the activity of this protein, which may keep cancer cells from growing.

watch and wait: A treatment plan that involves closely watching a patient's condition but not giving any treatment unless there are changes in test results that show the condition is getting worse. Watch and wait may be used to avoid or delay the need for treatments such as radiation therapy or surgery, which can cause side effects or other problems. During watch and wait, certain exams and tests are done on a regular schedule. Also called active surveillance.

will: A legal document that indicates who will receive a person's money and belongings and care for their children (if another parent can't) after death. If there is no will in place, an agent of the state may make these decisions.

X-ray: High-energy radiation that is used in low doses to provide images of the inside of the body and in high doses to treat cancer.

INDEX

NOTES

IMAGE CREDITS

Ten Tips for Living Well with Cancer (pages 8–9): Icons from The Noun Project, created by Adrien Coquet (steps), Jens Tärning (meditation), Gan Khoon Lay (teach), Guilherme Furtado (speech bubble), Eliricon (group), Colourcreatype (heart), Marie Van den Broeck (educate), Verry (handshake), P Thanga Vignesh (nutrition), and Zach Bogart (pencil)

Take a Break (page 88): Icons from The Noun Project, created by Adnen Kadri (sleep), Adrien Coquet (music; walk), Star and Anchor Design (television), Jens Tärning (meditation), Zach Bogart (pencil), BT Hai (movie), public domain (tennis), Adrien Coquet (restaurant), Pro-Symbols (tickets), and public domain (hiking)

In chapter 17: page 116, Kate Si/Shutterstock.com; page 117, zorina_larisa/Shutterstock.com; page 118, Kenishirotie/Shutterstock.com; page 119, Peteri/Shutterstock.com; page 120, Nataly Zhurakovski/Shutterstock.com

Recipe photography

Phytonutrient chart: hxdbzxy/Shutterstock.com (broccoli); Brent Hofacker/Shutterstock.com (prunes); Nitr/Shutterstock.com (blueberries/cherries); finchfocus/Shutterstock.com (carrots); gontabunta/Shutterstock.com (soybeans)

Fruit and Nut Bars: Elena Shashkina/Shutterstock.com

Quinoa Tabbouleh: YuliiaHolovchenko/Shutterstock.com

Pear and Blueberry Crumble: Anna Hoychuk/Shutterstock.com

Mixed Berry and Yogurt Crepes: Magdanatka/Shutterstock.com

Lemon Parmesan Chicken: Bondar Illia/Shutterstock.com

Kiwi Green Smoothie: tanjichica/Shutterstock.com

Shrimp Bento Bowl: SEAGULL_L/Shutterstock.com

White Fish Tacos: Eric Urquhart/Shutterstock.com

Swiss and Spinach Strata: nickichen/Shutterstock.com

Chocolate Mint Smoothie: Liliya Kandrashevich/Shutterstock.com

Chocolate Hummus: laran2/Shutterstock.com

Chocolate Hazelnut Spread: Allyso/Shutterstock.com

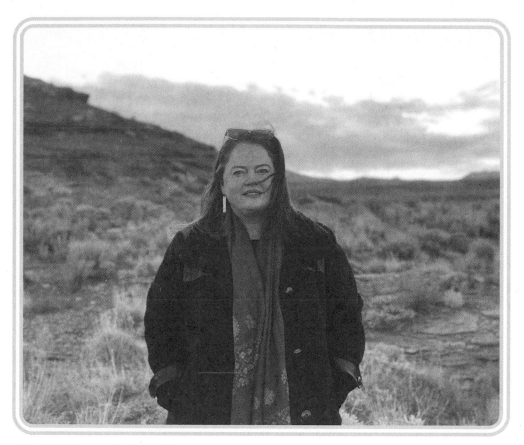

Kim Thiboldeaux on the Navajo Nation in Arizona.

ABOUT KIM THIBOLDEAUX

Executive Chair of the Cancer Support Community

As a nonprofit executive, thought leader, and author, **Kim Thiboldeaux** continues to make her mark on the global stage by ensuring that the patient's voice is at the center of every conversation about cancer.

Thiboldeaux served as CEO of the Cancer Support Community for more than twenty years, leading a global nonprofit network that operates at 175 locations, including CSC and Gilda's Club centers, and in multiple hospitals and cancer clinics. Combined with a toll-free helpline, educational materials, and digital platforms, this network of professionally led services provides more than $50 million each year in free support and navigation services to patients and families.

In 2019, Dr. Francis S. Collins, director of the National Institutes of Health, appointed Thiboldeaux to the Novel and Exceptional Technology and Research Advisory Committee. This panel is focused on providing advice and serves as a transparent forum for discussion of the scientific, safety, and ethical issues associated with emerging biotechnologies.

In June 2017, former vice president Joe Biden appointed Thiboldeaux to serve on the board of directors of the Biden Cancer Initiative (BCI). Thiboldeaux's service on BCI's board facilitated CSC's groundbreaking partnership with Airbnb. As a result of grants from Airbnb's Open Homes initiative, CSC has secured free housing valued at nearly $2 million for thousands of individuals in financial need who must travel for cancer treatment.

As part of Thiboldeaux's commitment to reach underserved communities, in May 2019 she joined Navajo Nation president Jonathan Nez, Dr. Jill Biden, hospital CEO Lynette Bonar, and leaders of the Tuba City Regional Health Care Corporation in Arizona to mark the opening of the first-ever full-time cancer care and support center on an American Indian reservation. After securing a generous gift from the Barbara Bradley Baekgaard Family Foundation, Thiboldeaux helped convene key Navajo Nation leaders, private sector supporters, and other officials to establish this culturally adapted program located in an area larger than the state of West Virginia.

In 2020, Stand Up to Cancer appointed Thiboldeaux to its Health Equity Breakthrough Research Team, focusing on cancers affecting underrepresented populations. In 2019, the International Psycho-Oncology Society presented her with its President's Community Award for Distinguished Contributions at its global congress in Canada.

Thiboldeaux's insights are highly sought after. She has been interviewed for the *Wall Street Journal*, the *Philadelphia Inquirer*, *Washington Post*, PBS, and WebMD, and her speaking engagements include a TEDx Talk and White House convenings. She is the author of *Reclaiming Your Life After Diagnosis*. Her writing is featured on *Medium* and in the *Huffington Post*.

A native of Philadelphia, Thiboldeaux grew up in a close-knit family of five children. In 2018, Thiboldeaux drove her father, a retired Philadelphia city bus driver and lifelong Eagles fan, to Minneapolis, where, together, they watched their beloved home team win its first Super Bowl title.

Thiboldeaux graduated from American University with a bachelor's degree in communications and a minor in Spanish. While at American, Thiboldeaux studied abroad in London and Buenos Aires, experiences that spurred her lifelong zest for travel. She has visited all seven continents, all fifty states, and fifty-plus countries around the world and has no intention of slowing down her exploration of new countries and cultures.